I0406804

# Sexually Transmitted Diseases – STDs

*A Valuable Resource for Sexual Good Health
for Teens, Adolescents, and Adults*

*Learn, Practice, Enjoy Safe Sex*

*Avoid Lethal Lure*

*By*

ARTHUR H.D'SOUZA PH.D.

(Front cover design adapted from CDC publication 99-8823)

ISBN: 1482780585
ISBN-13: 9781482780581

Library of Congress Control Number: 2013906490
CreateSpace Independent Publishing Platform, North Charleston, SC

This guide is designed to provide accurate information in regard to Sexually Transmitted Diseases. Transmission, symptoms, diagnosis, treatment, and management techniques are incorporated as an enabling framework for healthcare providers and readers. Constant changes, new improved procedures, and innovation of current practices may be at odds with prevailing knowledge and techniques therefore it's the sole responsibility of the practicing physician to deliver best care possible based on proven experience and knowledge.

Readers are strongly advised to seek and accept professional advice. Recommendations, procedures, products, and guidelines can assist readers to understand current choices available but only practicing physicians can advise, prescribe, and manage specific healthcare needs for patients.

Publishers, authors, and their representatives assume no liability for injury, damage, monetary or property loss arising out of recommendations, procedures, and products contained in this Guide.

# DEDICATION

Millions of women, young girls, boys, and children are sexually assaulted, mentally/physically abused, and exploited by predators and human traffickers. The barbaric practice is widespread in every part of the world but prevalent in most poor nations. Most victims are scarred for life if they ever survive the ordeal and very few somehow manage.

In my homeland, India, male child is preferred over baby girls. Clumsy reasons such as social/cultural or any other should not be a pretext to harm the newborn or the unborn. Female babies are marked for abortion regardless of term of pregnancy. Feticide of baby girls is condoned rather than punished in India. Innocent baby girls are abandoned, discarded like garbage, strangled, and even killed. Vanished victims out of mind, even professionals such as lawyers, medical personnel, police, and society at large hand in glove with abusive criminal parents ignore the problem. Even well-meaning social, religious, and political organizations play the proverbial three monkeys – "see nothing, hear nothing, and say nothing" therefore do nothing.

Abuse and exploitation of women and children is a serious problem worldwide. No reason, no amount of justification can be acceptable much less tolerated to ignore this scourge in our modern civil society. All countries, rich and poor have an obligation to protect all women and children (born and unborn) from predators and human traffickers. Stringent laws, tough penalties aside, much education, awareness, and greater commitment is urgently needed to eradicate this disgraceful menace. Protecting women and precious children should be everyone's top priority therefore every segment of civil society in every country must participate in this noble cause.

Many well - meaning kind hearted men and women, religious and non-religious affiliates spend much time and energy to bring hope and relief to many such victims. But much more needs to be done to make a difference for these desperate tender hearts.

## This Guide is dedicated to

Innocent children of all forms of abuse

Victims of mental and physical abuse

Victims of sexual abuse and exploitation

Kind, caring, compassionate healthcare givers worldwide

Concerned, dedicated community leaders, educators, religious leaders, and social activists

World leaders and champions of advocacy groups for children and less fortunate men and women

# ACKNOWLEDGEMENT

I am deeply grateful to my wife Margaret and our dear children Shaman and Shaz for the encouragement, help, and support I received throughout the preparation of this Guide. Their practical suggestions, valuable contribution, unlimited patience, and understanding made this project pleasant to accomplish.

Heartfelt thanks to Julie Sulfsted for cover design and selection of figures.

Cdre. Valentine Sequeira, whose unconditional valuable help and support is greatly appreciated.

Ameer Ullal for his superb computer support throughout the preparation of this manuscript.

Sincere thanks to my family, friends, and well-wishers for their generous help and continued support.

# CONTENTS

## Introduction

## Part I
### The Genital Anatomy

## Part II
### Sexually Transmitted Diseases of Viral Origin

## Part III
### Sexually Transmitted Diseases of Bacterial Origin

## Part IV
### Sexually Transmitted Diseases of Fungal, Bacterial, and Protozoan Origin

## Part V
### Sexually Transmitted Diseases by Parasites and Ectoparasites

## Part VI
### Violence against Women and Children

## Part VII

# Introduction

Everyone is acutely aware of influence and power of sex - that's the way it's been throughout history. Sex and sexual desires amongst us involve deeper personal feelings, intimacy, and biological need for procreation. Propagation of human race brings out the best of love and caring from us for future generations. It's a matter of pride to be a part of a process when our foot-prints matter. But enjoyable and rewarding sexual relationship can on occasions bring on undesirable consequences most of which can be avoided – this guide can be a useful tool for most such health conscientious persons.

Sexually transmitted diseases (STDs), a major health concern throughout the world are caused by pathogens that are transmitted by infected people through sexual activity. STDs are a result of pathogens entering new hosts, usually with greater virulence. The pathogens include bacteria, fungi, parasites, protozoans, and viruses. Most of the infectious agents are microscopic (bacteria and viruses), some are barely visible to the naked eye (itch mite), and few are large enough to be noticed (crabs and lice) on the skin or hair. Some STDs are nothing more than a nuisance, mere inconvenience, and discomfort but some can inflict great pain, life long suffering, and even death.

Sexually transmitted infections are very common in our modern society. An estimated 300 million people worldwide are presumed to be infected by one or more STDs. In the U.S. alone more than 3 million people are affected and the number is steadily growing. This trend is attributed to travel to any part of the world made easy, affordable, necessary, and also fun. This phenomenon has also contributed heavily to the spread of other diseases to millions worldwide. Socio/cultural acceptable behavior changes of last few decades have influenced attitude, customs, and social/family values. Universal access to social internet, real time communication, and increased friendship network has contributed heavily to cultural changes and attitude towards sex and sexuality. Some people believe these changes may have significantly contributed to factors such as:

- Increase in pre-marital sex.
- Decrease in age at which people engage in sexual intercourse.
- Social tolerance and acceptance of entertaining multiple sex partners.
- Increased divorce rate.

Sexually transmitted diseases, also known as Venereal Diseases (VDs) were named after the goddess of love and beauty Venus from Roman mythology. Until the 1940's only gonorrhea and syphilis were the recognized culprits. Dr. Paul Ehrlich (1854-1915), a German bacteriologist, discovered remedy for syphilis (Salvarsan) in 1910. Within a short time the miracle drug (antibiotic) Penicillin was isolated by British scientist, Alexander Fleming (1881-1955). This euphoric double blow was generally expected to wipe out sexually transmitted VDs but the excitement was short-lived. Gonorrhea and syphilis are still prevalent among sexually active men and women. Search for effective cure through research and other healthcare initiatives by developed countries have generated much interest and hope. In the process scientists have also discovered several other diseases acquired and transmitted by sexual activity. This guide deals with all such infections.

Education and greater awareness is essential to diagnose, treat, and prevent these serious infections. Even though sex is an important part of our life and future many social, religious, and cultural organizations do not promote sexual discourse. Rather than encourage open and honest discussion of sex and social impact of sexual behavior, many choose to turn a blind eye and a deaf ear in the hope that somehow the curious minds will not persist! Some openly discourage talk of sex. Some view sex as obscene, something to laugh at, joke, and ridicule. This attitude has developed strong moral, social, and cultural barrier in our daily lives. As a result, millions feel insecure, bothered, and confused by their innate sexual urges and desires.

People may get infected by any of the STDs for no fault of their own. Some may acquire STDs by accident or assault. Yet the society routinely rebukes such victims and worse patients are denied employment, healthcare, health insurance, housing, and other amenities. In most situations the stigma is hard to overcome. However the current welcome trend is to arrive at some acceptable standard and engage in useful, civil discourse. Meaningful and productive communication will benefit all concerned. The media, hand- in- glove with civic leaders and medical community have an obligation to educate and inform the public the facts, myths, consequences of unprotected sex, risks of sexual behavior, and benefits of safe sex.

Sexually transmitted infections are very common among most sexually active teens, adolescents, and adults. Modern medicine has identified more than 20 STDs. Some are painful, severe, and even fatal. Groups that are active transmitters of STDs are:

- Teen agers and adolescents.
- People who entertain multiple sex partners such as college students.
- Commercial sex workers (CSW).
- Alcoholics and needle sharing drug users.
- Prison population such as men and women doing time in correctional institutions.
- People living in crowded environments such as group homes, homeless shelters, slums, refugee camps, retirement communities, and dormitories.

Ever silent offending STDs can infect young adults, men, women of any age, socioeconomic, and educational background. Therefore medical community and media with active support from all sections of the society must engage in a public dialogue so the tide of infections can be reversed and eventually brought under control. Advantages and benefits of delivering accurate, reliable information versus consequences of misinformation must be made clear. Public awareness concerning practice of safe sex is critically important. Facts, myths, and fears of infection transmission, prevention, and control of STDs are also important deterrents in the fight to preserve and nurture a healthy society. It's possible to educate most adults and adolescents with the advanced instant communication systems at hand. The technological advances of medicine such as new devices, drugs, and medications can also be delivered to any part of the world with the existing air-speed and capacity.

STDs such as HIV, HPV, PID, and hepatitis can be fatal if not diagnosed and treated promptly. Some other STDs, especially herpes, gonorrhea, and chlamydia can be very painful with unpleasant adverse effects and severe complications. This book is designed to educate, inform, and bring much needed awareness concerning STDs to readers like you. The causative agents, mode of infection, symptoms, diagnosis, treatment, cure, prognosis, prevention and control are important factors that can help understand disease cycle fully. More you know better prepared you will be when faced with such misfortune. A list of most common misconceptions along with medically accurate information is made available so you may distinguish the truth from fiction. When in doubt, go to the nearest library or to your personal physician for reliable information. Don't risk your health – it's far too important that you enjoy good sexual health.

## Sexually Transmitted Diseases - Who is at Risk?

Even the most careful and diligent persons sometimes may find themselves embroiled in compromised locations, situations, and amongst people of questionable intent. Being aware of such situations is like winning the war before start of the battle against STDs. The following helpful facts are listed for your benefit - share them with people you love.

- Sexually transmitted infections are very common no matter which part of the world you go/ visit. Most tourist attractions may have a much higher rate of STDs.

- Teens and young adolescents are at the highest risk of contracting STDs. They are also soft targets and active dispensers of infections.
- People who entertain multiple sex partners such as teens and college students.
- Due to reasons of genital anatomy women are at a much higher risk of acquiring most common STDs than men.
- Millions of sex-workers and their patrons present a grave risk to society. Infected client's spouses and other contacts become innocent victims.
- Prison population, incarcerated adolescents and adults living in institutionalized setting such as group homes, correctional facilities, and prisons are at risk for acquiring and transmitting common STDs.
- People living in crowded environments such as dormitories, independent living, retirement communities, shelters for homeless, slums, and refugee camps are at much higher risk.
- Alcoholics and needle sharing drug addicts are at much greater risk for acquiring STDs.
- Sex toys and related paraphernalia sharing can increase risk for STDs.
- Pregnant women can infect the fetus in her womb and the baby at child birth.
- Uncircumcised men are more prone to STDs and other infections than their circumcised brothers.

- Victims (males, females, and children) of incest, rape, and sexual abuse are at much higher risk.
- All health care providers who come into contact with patient's blood, saliva, tissue, stool, and urine are at risk. Contaminated needles, surgical equipment, and all other soiled objects must be carefully handled.
- STDs can be transmitted by foreplay, fondling, touching, and kissing. Sexual penetration is not the only means of sharing germs.
- Spontaneous, unplanned, and unprotected sexual intercourse increases risk for common STDs.
- Infected asymptomatic persons can unknowingly transmit STDs.
- Some people (carriers) may be totally asymptomatic for life. Before you develop sexual intimacy with anyone confirm the disease status for the benefit of both of you.
- When possible relationship(s) become imminent, consult your health care provider. INSIST THAT BOTH OF YOU NEED BLOOD TEST AS A NEGATIVE CONFIRMATION. Your future partner and you need to feel safe. Good looks and noble intentions must be matched by deeds.

Health issues especially related to sexual activity are usually discussed only in classrooms for medical, premedical, nursing, and graduate students. These topics are a taboo in many places such as homes, private/ public functions, and parties. Sex related talk invites intense scorn and ridicule as such it is considered an embarrassment. Most people consider talk of sex and related issues strictly personal and private. Most youngsters however are willing to discuss issues related to sex - a welcome social change.

Feeling and touching genitals in public is considered offensive. This has greatly affected how most people generally behave even in private. Most adults do not examine their genitals routinely therefore fail to feel or discover any unusual lesions, blisters, or bumps. Most people if ever notice such bumps/sores usually ignore them in the hope that they may soon disappear. Vast majority of sexually active teens, young adults, and even mature adults are not familiar with the terms used to describe male and female sex organs or the genitals. The male and female reproductive systems are uniquely and functionally very different. The first chapter of this guide is devoted to introduce you to male and female genitals and the specific function (s) such organs perform. Such knowledge is necessary to understand normal and disease status of genitals. The vocabulary will help you correctly identify the part/organ that is affected or infected so you may communicate with your sex partner and also physician for better care.

## STDs – Communication

Sexually transmitted infections have been with us most likely throughout history, certainly as long as sex has been part of living, feeling self-gratification, and reproducing.

Yet ignorance about STIs leading to muted discussion, misinformation, and lack of accurate information has inflicted heavy loss of life and misery to so many for so long. Even the current generation for most part tactfully avoids discussion of sex and sex related matters for fear of ridicule. The general public, the religious groups, and multitude social organizations routinely treat issues of sex and sexually transmitted diseases with great disdain and much scorn. This attitude towards sexuality has prevented even the most socially active proponents of sex education to abstain from open discussion and sharing information with the most vulnerable members of our society - the curious teenagers. The media in general has taken a back seat for fear of repercussion, loss of revenue, and retribution. We must welcome issues that promote community health, human welfare, personal, and public hygiene for the greater good of all people and future generations. I suggest that civic, educational, political, and religious leaders in full cooperation with the medical community devise strategies to prevent, contain, and eradicate the scourge of sexually transmitted diseases for the greater good of general public and the millions infected with STDs. As we make accurate medical information available to the population at greatest risk and wipe out fictional myths and barriers, a measurable progress can be achieved. Parents, to-be parents, and guardians must accept their unique responsibility to communicate, inform, share, guide, and advise their prepubertal and pubertal children. The pros and cons, facts and fiction, and above all the benefits of having accurate information about sex and safe sexual activity dispensed by parents will make a greater impact on their darling children.

But then the parents and guardians also must be concerned over the reality that in the absence of parental discourse the youngsters will find such information somewhere else - the famous gutter. A list of falsehoods, convenient blind beliefs, and fictions with facts are provided for your serious consideration - test your knowledge.

## Sexually Transmitted Diseases - Facts or Fiction - You Decide

Modern society by design (?) has placed very serious obstacles for educators, health care providers, and even counselors to appropriately address, discus, and explain sex and sex related issues to teens and young adults. In the absence of heart to heart, frank, uninhibited dialogue, a vast majority of curious teens and young adults get their "answers" from their peers or wrong sources. For many sexually active teens and young adults this has created huge sea of confusion. They are unaware of facts, not know where to go and whom to trust. The convenient myths become a reality and way of life. A list of common disbeliefs may make your head spin. Some such myths commonly associated with sex are listed below.

- I feel great. I look good and healthy in the mirror. I have no lesions, swelling, and symptoms. I can't be infected.

Not True:

Looks can be deceiving. Many STDs such as hepatitis, herpes, HIV produce visual symptoms weeks or months after initial contact and in some individuals such symptoms may appear briefly and quickly disappear. Free of symptoms doesn't mean free of infection. Asymptomatic persons can infect sex partners.

- My friend and I are very careful. We play it safe all the time. Use new condoms and wash/clean after sex. We need not test for STDs. We cannot infect each other.

Not True:

You are not sure that your partner had history/exposure to STDs. Both of you may be symptom free for common STDs, worse yet you may be carriers. Condom covers only the penis. Skin to skin contact transmits infection. Hot/cold shower, genital wash after sex does not prevent common STDs.

- My partner and I have a true monogamous relationship. We are not promiscuous therefore will not acquire STDs.

Not True:

Current monogamous relationship doesn't guarantee that one of you have had no history or asymptomatic infection.

- Since my partner and I tested negative for STDs, we quit using condoms but wash with soap and hot water after sex.

Not True:

This doesn't prevent all infections all the time. Soap and hot water may reduce risk slightly but not completely for all common STDs.

- Healthy, active, young adults can fight off all STDs. They need not worry about additional protection.

Not True:
Anyone no matter how strong, healthy, and active can acquire common STDs.

- My partner and I practice only oral sex. It's safe, no condoms, and no worrisome sexually transmitted infections.

Not True:
STDs can be acquired via lesions, and tears in the mucous membrane in the mouth. Exchange of blood, saliva, and genital secretions can happen through broken skin.

- I had gonorrhea, chlamydia, and Trichomonas a few years ago. I will not get re-infected, I am immune.

Not True:
Bacterial, parasitic, and protozoan infections do not afford immunity like most viral infections.

- I can tell when someone has herpes by the outbreak: herpes sores and lesions on face and genitals. I abstain from sex until lesions disappear. The germs are transmitted only during viral outbreak.

Not True:
Outbreak or prodrome is neither a pre-requisite nor necessary to transmit herpes. Genital herpes can be asymptomatic in most people for a long time.

- My gynecologist gives me thorough annual check-up, blood, and pap tests. I am disease free.

**Not True:**
Good check-up is valid up to that point for some infections. Infections can go undetected by physical exams, pap-smear test, and blood tests. Antibodies may take months to appear in blood.

- My friends are free of STDs because they use condoms. I plan to protect myself like my friends do.

**Not True:**
Your friends have been fortunate. Condoms do not afford 100% protection to all STDs all the time. Condom covers only the penis. Skin to skin contact can infect partners during sex. Body fluids such as saliva, semen, and vaginal secretions may also readily cause infections.

# PART I
## The Genital Anatomy

### Male Reproductive System
### Female Reproductive System

A brief review of male and female reproductive systems is necessary to understand how diseases are sexually transmitted. Primary specific target for offending microbe (s), characteristic symptoms, and pathogenesis comprise disease/infection process. Males and females respond to variety of infectious agents differently due to sexual anatomical dissimilarities. This chapter describes male and female genital organs, their function, and result of an all-out infection.

## Male Reproductive System

Male genitals such as penis, scrotum, and testicles are located outside the body, quite a contrast to female genitals. Internal male reproductive organs include epididymis, vas deferens, seminal vesicle, prostate gland, and urethra. Not all STDs affect all organs. Some viruses such as HIV and hepatitis may not localize in the genitals but become systemic while most bacterial and protozoans may localize in one or more organs causing discomfort, pain, and discharge.

Genital organs are listed for learning convenience and not necessarily in any sequence of importance.

## Figure 1
### Male Reproductive Organs

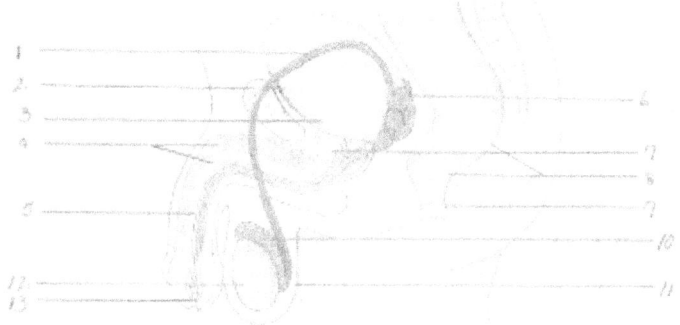

1. Vas deferens
2. Pubic bone
3. Urinary bladder
4. Erectile tissue: Corpora cavernosum and Corpus spongiosum
5. Penis
6. Seminal vesicle
7. Prostate gland
8. Large intestine
9. Rectum
10. Epididymus
11. Scrotum
12. Testicle
13. Urethral opening

## Penis:

Penis is a tube shaped fleshy organ. Average size of penis is between 6-8 inches but may vary from 4 – 9 inches for some. Penis has no bones or muscles, just three cylindrical tubes of spongy tissue, namely (a) corpus cavernosum x 2 and (b) corpus spongiosum x 1. Urethra, a hollow tube runs through corpus spongiosum and two corpus cavernosa side by side. Urethra carries urine from the bladder and semen with sperm during sexual intercourse (ejaculate) to the outside. Penis receives abundant blood supply via arteries and veins. Corpora cavernosa and corpus spongiosum get filled with blood upon sexual arousal. As a result penis becomes large, stiff, and erect. An erect penis can easily penetrate the vagina.

The end of penis, the glans or head is the most sensitive part due to numerous nerve endings around it. The head is usually stroked for penile arousal and orgasm that results in ejaculation. The glans in males is analogous to the female counterpart, the clitoris.

Most male newborns' penile head is covered with a thick layer of retractable foreskin or prepuce. Foreskin can be surgically removed days after birth - the procedure is known as circumcision. In most developed countries such as U. S. and Europe circumcision is performed days after child-birth. In some cultures and religions, a ritual is performed for this procedure either at child birth or at puberty. Circumcision is a safe procedure when performed by trained physicians. However males may suffer serious health issues if circumcised by untrained, unqualified persons under unsanitary, septic conditions.

Most healthcare providers and leading experts recommend circumcision for males. The procedure keeps the glans clean thereby preventing infection (s). Circumcised males have much lower rate of urinary tract infection than uncircumcised men. Risk of cancer, STDs such as HIV, herpes, other viral, bacterial, fungal (yeast), and protozoan infections are also lower among circumcised men. Uncircumcised men can repeatedly re-infect their partners as they carry pathogens between the glans and foreskin.

Some uncircumcised men may also develop a very painful penile discomfort called phimosis, a rare condition in which the foreskin tightens and will not retract. Cleaning, erection, ejaculation, and intercourse may become awkwardly painful. Surgical circumcision is the only option available to resolve phimosis.

Some cultures and ethnic groups in Africa and elsewhere practice a procedure called female circumcision. In this practice the clitoris and surrounding tissue is partially or completely removed. The procedure provides no benefits to female sexual health. In fact female genital mutilation can cause great discomfort, urogenital infection(s), and even death. Yet the practice still continues despite medical advice and strong objections from human rights activists.

## Scrotum:

Scrotum is a loose thin skinned wrinkled sac hangs just behind and below the penis. Scrotum contains two oval shaped testicles, right and left. The size and shape of testicles may vary from man to man. The enclosed testicles are provided with epididymis and vas deferens. Epididymis, a coiled tubule located on top of testis is the sperm reservoir. Epididymis collects sperm cells from the testis, allows sperm to mature, and move via vas deferens to the urethra. Vas deferens is a cordlike duct that carries sperm from the epididymis to seminal vesicles and prostate gland. Vas deferens tubules from right and left testicles meet at the back of the seminal vesicle and prostate gland. Prostate and seminal vesicles produce fluid that provides nourishment to sperm cells. This fluid constitutes bulk of the semen or the ejaculate. Semen containing sperm is expelled by the ejaculatory ducts to the outside during climax.

## Testicles:

Two enclosed testicles, hanging away and below the penis produce male hormone testosterone and sperm. Primary function of hormone testosterone is effecting growth and development of male physical characteristics. Testicles require lower temperature (than the body) to produce sperm cells that are eventually stored in the epididymis. Sperm cells are ejaculated into the cervix during intercourse. Sperms move rapidly, find the egg (s), penetrate, and fertilize to initiate conception.

Testicular cancer though rare, is a concern for young men. Therefore all adolescents and men must routinely self - examine their testicles periodically. If unusual bumps appear associated with pain and irritation, see your physician immediately. Testicular cancer and/or severe orchitis may cause sterility in men. Orchitis, infection of testicles is caused by mumps virus.

## Internal Male Reproductive Organs
## Epididymis:

Epididymis is analogous to a spindle. It consists of long coiled tubules that store newly formed sperm cells and allow them to mature. Mature sperms are then transported by the vas deferens to the seminal vesicles and prostate gland.

Chlamydia and gonorrhea are most common infections of epididymis causing scrotal pain and swelling. Epididymitis is a STD that must be treated promptly.

## Vas Deferens:

Vas deferens tubules from right and left testicles bring mature sperm cells to seminal vesicles and prostate gland. The fluid produced by the seminal vesicles and prostate gland along with sperm that constitutes semen is then expelled by the ejaculatory ducts. The nerves, blood vessels, along with each vas deferens form the spermatic cord.

When friction on the glans is at heightened stimuli, nerves initiate strong muscle contractions along the ducts of the epididymis, vas deferens, the seminal vesicles, and the prostate gland. These powerful contractions force semen into the urethra. Muscles around the urethra contract as well, thus semen is propelled through and out of the penis.

Men who desire no (more) children get their vas deferens surgically cut. The procedure is called vasectomy.

## Prostate Gland and Seminal Vesicles:

Prostate gland is located just below the bladder in the pelvis and firmly surrounds the mid portion of the hollow urethra. The normal healthy prostate gland is no bigger than the size of a walnut. Usually prostate gland enlarges with age, inflammation, infection, and in men with prostate cancer. When this occurs, urination, intercourse, and other sexual activity may become extremely painful. The seminal vesicles lie just above the prostate glands. The prostate and the seminal fluids that nourish sperm is a major component of semen, the ejaculate that vas deferens carries to the urethral opening and to the outside. The thick viscous fluid (semen) consists of sperm, prostatic fluid, seminal fluids, and the fluids from vas deferens.

Disease, inflammation, and infection of the prostate are very common among men of advanced age. Prostate cancer is found in 50 percent of men over age 70 and among almost all men aged over 90. Most of these disorders rarely manifest or cause symptoms due to slow progression of the cancer itself. Yet in some men, for unknown reasons cancer grows and spreads much faster. Sexually transmitted infection of prostate is very rare but may occur if urethral infection is not treated promptly.

## Urethra:

Urethra is a hollow tubule that has dual function. It carries urine from the bladder to the outside of the body and expels semen (as described above) during sexual activity.

Most sexually transmitted infections (STIs) caused by bacteria, yeast, virus, and protozoans often affect urethra. When infected, urethra will burn, itch, and exude pus cells along with blood. Urination, masturbation, and intercourse may become excruciatingly painful.

## Female Reproductive System

Unlike male genitals, most of the female reproductive organs are located inside the abdominal cavity. External and internal female genital organs are described below.

## External Genital Organs – Vulva

External female genital organs such as labia majora, labia minora, and clitoris are collectively called vulva. The anatomy of the vulva shown below is distinctly different than that of male genitals. Two important functions of the vulva are:

1. Protect internal reproductive organs from pathogens and harmful foreign objects.
2. Admit sperm to fertilize egg(s) for reproduction.

## Labia majora and labia minora:

Labia majora or large lips are relatively large, smooth, and fleshy. The tender lips extend from the prepuce (top of the clitoris) to the introitus (vaginal opening). As girls reach puberty the labia majora develops pubic hair. Fatty oil secreting sweat and sebaceous glands are located on the labia majora.

Labia minora, the small fleshy pink lips lie just below the large lips and cover urethral/vaginal openings. Labia majora and labia minora together provide a barrier to pathogens and opportunistic microbes from entering urethra, vaginal canal, and cervix. Internal organs can get infected usually by intercourse, sexual activity, or self- infliction such as douching. Most infections can produce visible symptoms on the vulva, cervix, urethra, vaginal canal, and other internal genital organs. Some infections may be limited to vulva but most affect internal genitals.

## Figure 2
### External Genital Organs – Vulva

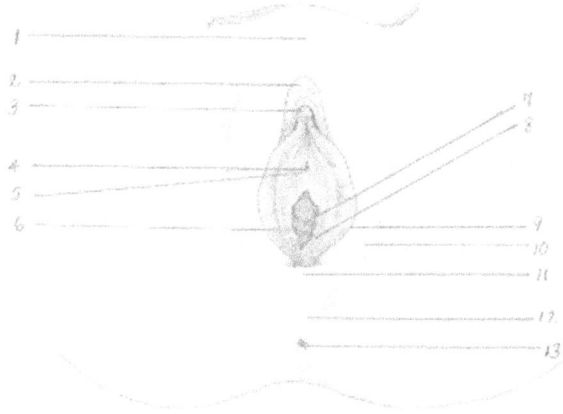

1. Mons pubis      2. Prepuse – Foreskin
3. Clitoris      4. Urethral opening (Urinary opening)
5. Skene's glands      6. Hymen - Maidenhead
7. Vaginal opening (Orifice or Introitus)
8. Bartholin's gland      9. Labia minora
10. Labia majora      11. Fourchette
12. Perineum      13. Anus

## Clitoris:

The labia minora lips (right and left) meet at the bottom of the clitoris. Clitoris is a small protrusion analogous to the penis but for size. The prepuce (foreskin) that covers the clitoris is very similar to penile foreskin. Clitoris is very sensitive to stimulation and functionally comparable to the penile head in men. Like the glans, clitoris is highly sensitive to stimuli. Sexual arousal followed by climax improvised by clitoris just like the glans in men.

## Internal Female Genital organs

Internal female genital organs function efficiently from the time sperm enter the cervix until child-birth. These organs form the genital pathway starting from the ovaries down to vaginal canal. The sperm propelled during intercourse can only move up the genital tract and eggs flow down the pathway (tract) as described below.

- Ovaries release eggs through the fallopian tubes (oviducts) for fertilization.
- Eggs meet sperm in the oviduct for fertilization.
- Fertilized egg (embryo) moves down to attach to the uterine wall.
- Embryo develops into fetus (baby).
- Fully developed baby exits mothers' womb through vaginal canal.

# Figure 3
## Internal Female Genital Organs

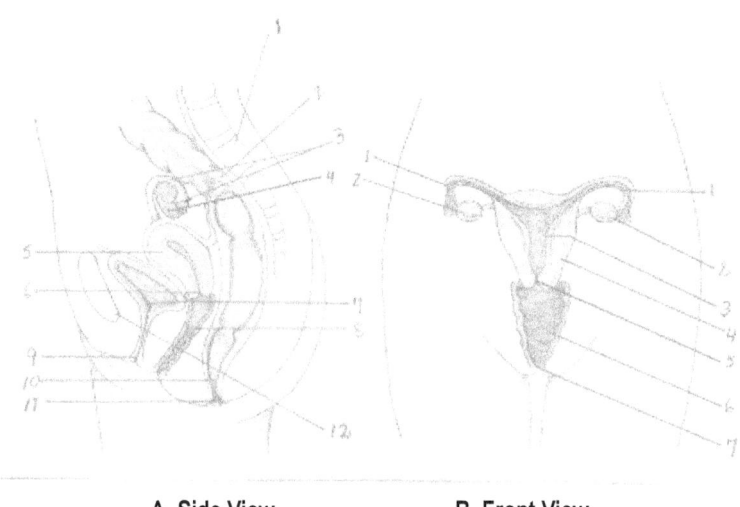

A. Side View          B. Front View

| | | |
|---|---|---|
| 1. Backbone | 2. Large Intestine | 1. Fallopian Tubes |
| 3. Fallopian Tube | 4. Ovary | 2. Ovaries |
| 5. Uterus | 6. Cervix | 3. Endometrium |
| 7. Bladder | 8. Vaginal canal | 4. Uterus |
| 9. Urethra | 10. Rectum | 5. Cervix |
| 11. Anus | 12. Pubic bone | 6. Vaginal canal |
| | | 7. Vaginal opening |

## Vagina and Bartholin's Glands:

The vaginal mouth is covered by front and back tissues or walls. It can be easily opened for examination and inter-course. Vaginal cavity/canal is a muscular structure that is 3 to 4 inches long in pubertal women. Hymen (maidenhead) usually completely covers the vaginal opening in a virgin. Hymen membrane may tear at attempted intercourse or other form of force. The muscles of lower part of the vagina help control its diameter while upper muscles (just below cervix) can be easily stretched during examination or sexual activity. Cervix, mouth, and neck of uterus are located at the top of the vaginal canal.

A clear odorless discharge due to shedding of mucosal cells of vaginal wall is normal for most women. Vaginal canal may harbor lactobacilli and yeast that are non-pathogenic. Sexually active women can acquire infections of bacterial, fungal, protozoan, and viral origin from infected partners.

A pair of tiny pea shaped glands - the Bartholin's glands are located just below the vaginal opening on each side. These glands provide thick lubricants (secretions) during intense sexual intercourse. Gonorrhea, chlamydia, yeast, and host of other pathogens can cause vaginal infections. Bartholin's and Skene's glands (located on each side of the Urethra) can also get infected, swollen, and intensely painful.

## Cervix:

Cervix is located just below the uterus at the top of the vaginal canal. Women can feel their cervix for self- examination. The opening of the cervix (to the uterus) known as Oz has dual functions.

- Oz allows menstrual blood to flow out during menstrual cycle (period).
- Admits sperm into the uterus/fallopian tubes to meet egg (s) for fertilization.

Cervix can acquire bacterial, fungal, protozoan, and viral infections. Cervical cancer and genital warts by human papillomavirus (HPV) is a grave concern for girls and women of all ages. Regular gynecological examinations and pap- smear tests are a must for all sexually active and not so active females.

## Uterus - The Womb:

Uterus is a pear-shaped pouch like organ that sits upside down behind the bladder in front of the rectum and on top of the vagina. This is where the fertilized egg, the embryo starts to grow into fetus. Uterus receives generous supply of blood for nourishment and continued development of the embryo.

Uterus consists of corpus (main body) and cervix, the lower part. Corpus is a highly muscular organ that can enlarge to hold the growing fetus during the entire term of pregnancy. The muscular walls contract during labor to force (push) baby through the stretched fibrous cervix down through the vaginal canal.

Inner wall of the corpus, the endometrium thickens after menstruation in anticipation of conception. If the woman does not fertilize (get pregnant) during this cycle, bulk of the endometrial cells will be shed during menstrual period.

## Ovaries and Fallopian Tubes (Oviducts):

Most women have two (right & left) pearl colored oval shaped ovaries that are analogous to male testicles. The size of an ovary is about 3 to 4 cm across or slightly smaller than a hard-boiled egg. Ovaries produce female hormones: estrogen and progesterone. Most women of child-bearing age (normally up to age 45) release an egg at the middle of the menstrual cycle. The egg falls into the opening of the funnel shaped end of the fallopian tube. The egg is then propelled by cilia (hair like protrusions) and inner muscle lining of the fallopian tube's wall downward. If the egg encounters sperm in the fallopian tube fertilization can occur- result is a tiny embryo. Embryo moves slowly while the embryonic cells continue to divide and multiply. Embryo eventually reaches the uterus and gets embedded to the uterine wall. This process is called implantation - the beginning of a normal pregnancy.

Sometimes fertilized egg is unable to travel down to the uterus due to obstacles such as inflammation, infection, scarring, and obstruction in the fallopian tubes. This abnormal process known as ectopic or tubal pregnancy is a serious medical emergency. In an ectopic pregnancy embryo grows in the fallopian tube (s) causing intense pressure, internal bleeding, and eventual rupture that may be fatal.

Almost all internal genital organs can be infected by STDs. Victims of pelvic inflammatory disease (PID) caused by multiple opportunistic bacteria and other agents endure chronic pain and discomfort in the abdomen and pelvis.

## Urethra and Skene's glands:

Urine is carried from the bladder to the outside via urethra. The urethral opening is located just below the clitoris. Skene's glands on each side of the urethra secrete lubricating fluid to the vagina during sexual stimulation.

Urethral and bladder infections (UTI) are more common in women than men. Most sexually transmitted diseases also infect urethra, Skene's glands, and bladder. These infections can itch, burn, and make urination very painful. To avoid greater discomfort and severe complications promptly see your physician when these symptoms appear.

# PART II
## Sexually Transmitted Diseases of Viral Origin

## 1. Acquired Immune Deficiency Syndrome - AIDS Human Immunodeficiency Virus Infection – HIV

Human immunodeficiency virus, a retrovirus is the cause of this very complex and incurable disease. Once rare, AIDS is very common among teens, adults, and even children worldwide. Reports of the disease in the early 1980's caused near panic conditions, alarmed medical community, and received attention from world leaders. AIDS epidemic of the 1990's has claimed millions of lives worldwide as it peaked in 1999. Today, in the U.S. alone someone is infected with HIV every nine and a half minutes. Worldwide incidence rate of this dreadful disease is a cause of great concern for everyone. December 1, is designated world AIDS day to remember victims of AIDS and bring awareness to all.

HIV causes slow depletion of white blood cells also known as CD4 cells and aggressively destroys body's immune system thus exposing the host to a variety of health issues and fatal opportunistic infections. As a result immune compromised host acquires immunodeficiency syndrome (AIDS). Patients eventually succumb to opportunistic infections and certain types of cancers. AIDS is the last stage of dreadful HIV infection that is usually fatal.

HIV/AIDS affects mostly young adults. In the western hemisphere most of the initial victims were homosexual men. Drug users by needle injection were also equally affected. However the rate of infection and transmission has steadily increased among heterosexual men and women in recent years. Thousands of children born to infected mothers acquire HIV while still in the womb. Blood transfusion was also a source of transmission but improved testing has minimized risk for HIV. Yet for many children and victims of sexual/physical abuse HIV is a real threat.

There are two virus types that cause HIV/AIDS, HIV- I and HIV - 2. HIV- type I is prevalent worldwide and HIV - 2 is mostly found in West Africa. Many people infected by HIV -2 are also already infected with HIV -I. Therefore most clinics and laboratories in the U.S. and world over include Type I and 2 for testing purposes.

Infection and transmission of the virus is usually associated with a person's social and sexual behavior. Victims' age, color, race, ethnicity, education, social status, and sexual preference are hardly a matter of debate. Risk for acquiring HIV is higher   with unsafe sex so is infected blood via blood transfusion (s) and needle sharing. HIV is transmitted by body fluids such as blood, saliva, semen, and vaginal secretions of infected people.  Other body fluids such as breast milk, cerebrospinal fluid, tears, and urine may also contain HIV particles but at much lower concentrations.

## Transmission:

- Most people acquire HIV from infected sex partners. Transmission can occur by infected body fluids such as semen, saliva, and vaginal secretions that contains virus.

- Unprotected genital-oral, anal/oral, and vaginal/anal sex can transmit HIV.
- Foreplay can be risky. HIV positive sex partners can transmit the virus by fluid exchange.
- Breaks or cuts in the mucous membrane, the protective lining of the mouth, rectum, urethra, and vagina facilitate virus entry into susceptible host. The virus will then enter the blood stream and target CD4 cells.
- Transfusion of contaminated whole blood, plasma, and blood products has resulted in HIV infections. However such infections are rare in the U.S. and elsewhere since 1985. At present most countries process and screen blood and blood products for HIV type I and 2 routinely.
- Needle sharing by drug users, a very common practice can transmit HIV. Needle sharing by drug addicts has subsided to some degree since HIV infection peaked in the 1990's. Yet the practice has not completely stopped.
- Accidental needle sticks, contact with infectious body fluids, tissue, and other tainted objects can also transmit HIV.
- Surgical staff, nursing staff, phlebotomists, IV Therapists, and all health care providers are always at risk of acquiring HIV infection. Even though many safety procedures are in place accidents can still happen.

- Infected pregnant women and mothers are a high risk to newborns. This can happen before or during natural child-birth and also through breastfeeding.
- Studies have shown that infections such as herpes, syphilis, and other common STDs predispose persons for HIV infection.

## Prevention of HIV Transmission:

- Total abstinence is the safest way to live HIV free.
- Have sex with only HIV free partner who has strictly monogamous relationship with you and of course you maintain the same.
- Always practice safe sex. Consider barriers such as male/female condom, rectal, and vaginal microbicides. Talk to your doctor for best option.
- Avoid spontaneous sex and sex with persons of unknown STD history.
- Avoid sex with alcoholics and needle sharing drug addicts.
- Avoid sex with commercial sex workers (CSW).
- Avoid other STDs. Most STDs predispose sexually active persons to HIV.
- Pre-exposure and post exposure prophylaxis is also a recommended preventive tool. Healthcare professionals, victims of sexual assault and abused children can benefit from this treatment option.
- Consider circumcision – procedure is safe at any age.

- Cold/hot shower, washing genitals, and urination after sex will not prevent HIV and other common STDs.

## HIV Infection – Myths

As AIDS epidemic spread and peaked in the 1990s, so did fear and myths. Contrary to claims and widespread belief, HIV does not spread nor infect people by:

- Casual or social contact with an infected person such as shaking hands, hugging, and other forms of non-sexual physical contact.
- Sharing living quarters, clothes, work place, classroom, public or private toilet, shower, and water fountain are risk free so is sharing food, drink, and refreshments.
- HIV/AIDS patient cannot infect others by breathing, sneezing, and coughing in "your airspace".
- Dog bite, cat scratch, insect bite, and other animals may cause infection but NOT HIV.
- Donating and receiving blood, kidney, and other organs is safe. The sterile techniques, disposable needles, and greater awareness among healthcare community has done it.
- Handling fecal matter, urine, saliva, and drainage of wounds in a clinic, medical facility, or nursing home requires skill and extreme care. Though HIV is not a threat, adequate care and precaution must be exercised when handling such matter. Better be safe than sloppy and sorry.

- Healthcare professionals receive instruction and on the job training in the U.S. All new and current employees are required to attend OSHA work - shops to learn safe health care practices.
- Victims of rape and sexual assault are at great risk. When faced with such a situation take courage, do not panic but get professional help – sooner the better. Current advances in treatment and management can help prevent HIV/AIDS.
- Dirty rest rooms and toilet seats are repulsive yet cause no HIV or STDs.
- HIV transmission from dentist/physicians to patients is rare. Since the advent of HIV epidemic health care providers in the U. S. take additional precautions and play it safe.

## Life Cycle of Human Immunodeficiency Virus

Life cycle for HIV begins when it enters the host and attaches itself to the protein coat - cell wall of target cell, the CD4 lymphocyte. CD4 lymphocytes are critical part of immune system. The virus takes over the genetic machinery of CD4 lymphocyte(s) destroying them in the process. HIV reproduces in great numbers by repeating the cycle. Critical enzymes - protease, integrase, and reverse transcriptase facilitate HIV life cycle in CD4 lymphocyte. Recent medical advances have produced drugs that block, inhibit, mimic, neutralize, or destroy viral enzyme activity thus provide suppressive and prophylactic advantage to millions of patients worldwide. Victims of abuse, sexual assault, rape, and incidental/accidental exposure to HIV also can greatly benefits from these newer drugs.

## Figure 4
### CD4 Lymphocyte

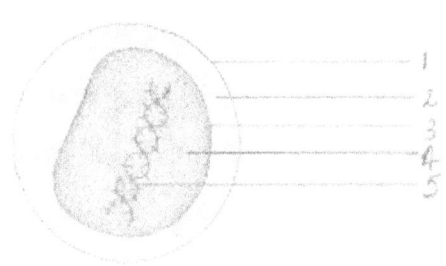

1. Cell Wall
2. Cytoplasm
3. Nuclear membrane

4. Nucleus
5. Cell DNA

## Figure 5 A
### HIV Virus Attachment and New Virus Formation

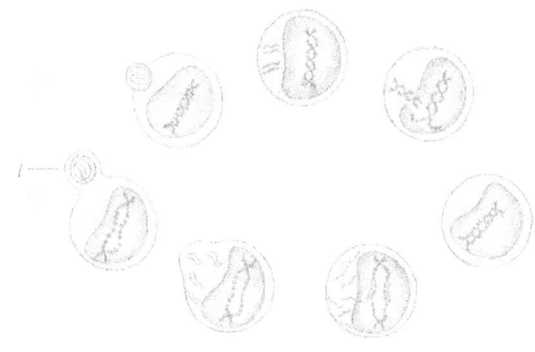

1. Newly formed virus budding away from CD4 cell

## Figure 5 B
### Newly Formed Mature Viruses ready to infect CD4 Cells

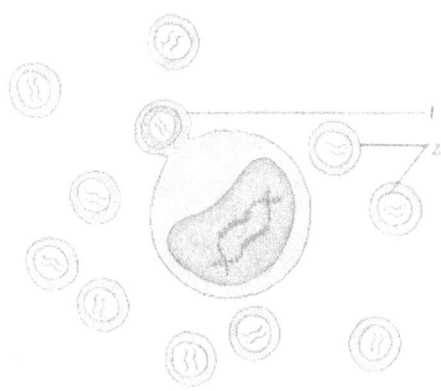

1. Newly formed immature virus
2. Mature virus ready to infect CD4 cells

Life Cycle of HIV as described below is an ongoing process in the host. Each cycle may produce hundreds of new virus.

1. HIV attaches to receptor site on CD4 lymphocyte. This initial binding step is facilitated by enzymes produced by the virus.
2. Virus fuses with the cell wall and penetrates CD4 cell.
3. RNA, the genetic material of the virus is released into CD4 cell.
4. Enzyme Reverse Transcriptase converts HIV RNA into viral DNA.
5. Newly formed viral DNA integrates with CD4 cell's DNA facilitated by viral enzyme integrase.

6. Resulting DNA replicates and produces small bits of RNA and long protein chains by a process known as transcription via enzyme Transcriptase.
7. Bits of RNA and protein are assembled by enzyme Protease into hundreds of new immature virus particles inside the host cell.
8. Immature virus burst open the host cell membrane, get covered by a piece of protein coat in the process and mature.
9. More viruses are ready to repeat the infectious cycle as described above. Increased virus population (load) circulating in the host destroys CD4 cells. Immune system is thus effectively "knocked out" predisposing patients to other potentially life threatening opportunistic infections and malignancies.

Most AIDS patients (worldwide) were homosexual men who acquired the dreadful disease by having sex with other men. In the U.S. and world over this generated some degree of scorn, distaste, and social stigma for victims of AIDS. Infected persons were wary of seeking medical aid, treatment, and counseling for fear of discrimination, ridicule, and rejection. When AIDS epidemic was in its early stages in the 1980s, and early 1990s, people infected with HIV were denied usual and customary amenities, health insurance, jobs, and housing. Fear of harassment, rejection, and denial of common services prevented people from "coming out" to seek and receive proper care. As a result many victims of AIDS silently died.

Although initial AIDS victims were mostly homosexual men and women, heterosexual activity is most dreaded mode of transmission of HIV at present. Like many viral diseases, HIV infection in most people may be totally asymptomatic. Infected people may be symptom free for months and years hence can unknowingly transmit HIV to their sex partners. Therefore it's critically important that people seek prompt medical advice when confronted with slightest suspicion of HIV infection. Appropriate care, counseling, and follow-up treatment may produce favorable outcome if professional help sought promptly.

## Symptoms for HIV:

Most people usually do not develop symptoms that are truly characteristic of the disease. However many newly infected people may experience some or all of the symptoms listed below.

- Some people may experience symptoms similar to those for infectious mononucleosis, a common infection among teens and young adults.
- Many develop flu-like symptoms such as fatigue, fever, sore throat, headache, muscle aches, nausea, and vomiting.
- Swollen lymph nodes in the arm pits, groin, and neck may be itchy and painful.
- Lack of appetite, anxiety, restlessness, and general discomfort are also common.
- Some people may develop red rash over the entire body or parts of the body.
- Symptoms may resolve with no treatment within a few weeks. Most victims may not suspect HIV infection therefore seek no help.

Newly infected persons usually go through an initial asymptomatic phase known as latent or dormant phase. This is when most people develop antibodies in response to HIV infection, also known as seroconversion. Large amounts of virus circulate in the blood and body fluids of infected persons who become contagious to sex partners. Some people may remain asymptomatic for a long time but be contagious. Most such people may repeatedly experience mild to moderate symptoms but symptoms may resolve within days therefore unaware of their infection.

Seroconversion process is host's response to the invading virus that is foreign to the host. Host produces antibodies (proteins) to combat specific virus threat, in this case HIV. Circulating HIV destroy host's CD4 cells, causing a drop (decline) of CD4 cell count. As the number of CD4 cells decline so will the body's ability to fight numerically superior viral onslaught. When CD4 cell count falls below 200 cells per microliter of blood, characteristic symptoms of the disease become obvious. Recommended criteria to confirm HIV is when CD4 count is less than 50 cells per microliter of blood. Normal CD4 count is more than 500 cells per microliter of blood. Distinctive symptoms of full blown HIV/AIDS to support definitive diagnosis include:

- Swollen, painful lymph nodes all over the body.
- Rashes, bruises, lesions, and sores that will not heal.
- Sudden, unexplained weight loss or a wasting syndrome, loss of appetite, memory loss (dementia), weakness of arms, and legs.

- Off and on fever, cough, shortness of breath, and an un-well feeling.
- Profuse night sweats.
- Anemia, fatigue, and restlessness.
- Chronic headache, anxiety, and depression.
- Frequent and recurring diarrhea.
- Persistent thrush in the mouth and genital (yeast) infection.
- Recurring opportunistic infections of bacterial, fungal, protozoan, and viral origin.
- Kaposi's sarcoma and non-Hodgkin's lymphoma may also develop.

An infected person's immune system from get go fights back and usually succeeds to keep the body infection free but HIV out-smarts body's defense system by destroying CD4 cells that are necessary to fight and neutralize the invading virus. Weakened immune system now becomes more vulnerable to attacks from several opportunistic organisms, that were until now caused no harm. Recurring cold, fever, nausea, diarrhea, and several other disabling episodes eventually cause immune system failure. People with HIV/AIDS are highly susceptible and become ideal targets for opportunistic infections of bacterial, fungal, protozoan, and viral origin. Pneumococcal pneumonia, tuberculosis, shingles (herpes zoster), yeast infection, Kaposi's sarcoma, non-Hodgkin's lymphoma, several other forms of ailments, cancers, and malignancies are most common opportunistic infections that affect HIV/AIDS victims. As CD4 cell count declines further, more serious and complex ailments develop resulting in fatalities.

Most symptoms listed above presumed to be caused by HIV. In fact these are likely to be due to one or more opportunistic infections. Your physician can best explain why certain symptoms persist and possibly suggest remedies to you. Develop a list of all symptoms in the order they appeared as you prepare to visit your doctor. Note the day and time such symptoms first appeared and reappeared. Symptoms may be different for men and women. Some symptoms may be age related. Not all patients experience all symptoms all the time.

## Diagnosis:

Even a faintest suspicion of probable HIV infection can be devastating to say the least. No matter how strong you are (mentally and physically), very chance of exposure to HIV risk may make you angry, fearful, upset, and distraught. However it's wise to think ahead, plan your next move, and prepare to face reality. One would hope to get the good news, yet knowing the truth so you may face the facts sooner than later may bring you greater comfort through timely medical intervention and appropriate care.

Most healthcare providers in the U.S. have the knowledge and experience to detect and diagnose HIV infection. Medical services and care are provided with utmost urgency. Personal and medical information is collected with patients' privacy and dignity in mind therefore prospective patients must provide confidential details related to presumed exposure to HIV including current symptoms. Healthcare providers must be made aware of circumstances, number of sexual encounters including number of sex partners (if more than one), or people sharing needles at the time.

Other forms of exposures such as physical/sexual abuse are also critical for diagnosis and follow-up care.

Based on your presentation and physical examination your physician may request stool, urine, and sputum samples. Genitals may be swabbed and discharge sent for laboratory analysis. Blood tests for HIV antibody and antigen will be made. Liver function tests to determine liver damage are also critical for diagnosis. In some unusual cases physician (s) may even request more definitive, sophisticated, and expensive blood tests. Most likely negative results will bring you much anticipated relief. This experience should also remind you to exercise greater care in partner selection, alcohol/drug use, adjusting behavior, needle sharing, and safe sex practices for your protection and peace of mind.

Your physician may also request tests for other common STDs such as chlamydia, gonorrhea, hepatitis (B&C), herpes, HPV, syphilis, and others. Based on patient history CD4 lymphocyte count, HIV plasma viral load analysis, tests for opportunistic infections such as toxoplasma, tuberculosis, and others may be requested.

## Testing for HIV - Confidentiality Issues:

Clinics, laboratories, and doctor's offices are well equipped to perform test (s) for HIV. All such tests are performed in strict confidence. Usually a small amount of venous blood is secured, labeled appropriately (no name only number) for identification and testing purposes. On occasion an oral swab is also obtained and tested. The entire testing and verification process may take weeks or longer - a dreaded waiting period.

Almost all HIV testing, regardless of your personal reasons must be done confidentially and anonymously. The procedure is for your peace of mind and not for your professional/career advancement therefore you must take precautions that such procedure(s) do not become part of your medical record and history. Almost all states in the U.S. have laws to protect patient's privacy.

## HIV Antibody Test:

Most HIV infected people develop antibodies in response to HIV within 8-12 weeks post exposure. In some persons positive antibody detection may take much longer. Antibody test (s) can be performed for HIV-I or HIV-2 on body fluids such as blood, saliva, and vaginal secretions. Routine antibody tests at times can be misleading due to unknown reasons or insufficient quantity of specific antibodies in patients' blood at the time. The test may be repeated 4-6 weeks after the initial test for definitive results. In most situations additional more sensitive tests may also be requested.

## EIA and Western Blot Tests:

EIA - Enzyme Immunoassay is accurate and sensitive. Occasionally false positive (due to interference) or negative result may be reported by a testing facility. Healthcare providers may suggest much more sensitive, reliable, and expensive Western blot test (Immunofluorescence assay) to confirm original findings. Western blot assay identifies specific antibodies to HIV antigens such as protein p24, gp41, and gp120/160. However like the EIA test, Western blot assay also requires up to six months to be accurate. In some extreme rare cases, repeat EIA and Western blot tests are recommended at 3 and 6 month interval for persons with rare immune disorders who may not produce detectable quantities of antibodies (as normal people) in time for convenient testing.

## HIV Antigen Test:

HIV antigen assay is sensitive and reliable. If and when virus gains entry into a host the protein (antigen) fights off body's defenses, the immune system. The specific component of the protein that attacks/stimulates the immune system for HIV is identified as p24. The test is called p24 antigen test. Ideally p24 antigen test can be routinely used to detect all new infections. But in the initial stages of HIV infection viral concentration in the body is relatively low therefore a definitive result is questionable. As the infection progresses due to viral multiplication, antigen concentration also increases. At this point antibody test is recommended because it's convenient, reliable, expedient, and above all highly cost effective than p24 test.

P24 antigen test is routinely used to screen all blood donors who may be infected    but not yet developed antibodies to HIV. This is a sense of relief to all blood recipients. Another advantage of p24 antigen test is in screening infants born to HIV infected mothers. Most of these newborns will have detectable levels of antibodies also. Presence of p24 antigen in the infant is an indication and confirmation of HIV infection. P24 antigen test is highly recommended for victims of all forms of sexual assault, physical abuse and accidental/incidental exposure. Experts recommend that all victims of sexual assault, especially abused children be tested for p24 antigen for medical, legal, and prophylactic considerations.

It is important to point out that HIV/AIDS is a very complex disease. There are no simple solutions, yet some of the following suggestions may help. But not all suggestions are for everyone and not everyone must follow all suggestions – different situations require different solutions therefore patients must consult their physician and develop best options for their unique condition.

- When you suspect that you may have been infected, call your healthcare provider or clinic to make an appointment – do not procrastinate.
- Describe in detail how you may have acquired HIV.
- Make sure that your healthcare provider is knowledgeable and understands your situation fully. This may be difficult at first yet based on your experience you must decide if he/she can guide you appropriately. Good communication with your physician is critically important for your very survival.
- Based on your symptoms (if any yet) and history you may be advised to take EIA/ Western blot tests, p24 antigen test, or antibody test.
- If tests are negative, your healthcare provider may seek a repeat in 4-6 weeks from the last test. This may be done as a precautionary measure.
- Your healthcare provider may also suggest tests and procedures for other STDs. Your current disease status and the extent of damage to your immune system and vital organs need to be evaluated.

- Your experienced healthcare provider has a good road map and sound advice for your good health. When not sure or have concerns consider talking to him/her. Get all your questions answered.
- While going through treatment (if positive) or having the comfort of being not infected, find helpful literature in your local library to stay informed of latest developments about HIV/AIDS. Most communities, libraries, and schools also offer much instruction, information, and guidance free of charge.

## Treatment:

HIV infection is very complex. Retroviral syndrome requires sophisticated multi-prong approach from get go. HIV can begin with a brief acute infection but without prompt treatment may progress into full blown AIDS and eventual death. Therefore early detection and timely intervention is critical. Treatment and management of AIDS is a unique medical challenge for healthcare providers. Most healthcare providers in the U. S. are well aware of latest techniques, treatment options, and effective drugs to fight HIV. Improved HIV/AIDS management techniques, counseling by supportive staff has also resulted in favorable outcome. Based on patient's disease status physicians may suggest and execute the following treatment procedure (s).

- Recommend restoring immune system by timely intervention.
- Help increase CD4 cell count while lowering viral load with medications.

- Recognize, anticipate, prevent, also treat, and cure opportunistic infections.
- Evaluate previous and current STDs, hepatitis A, B, & C status, and suggest resolution.
- Propose behavioral changes and offer emotional and psychological counseling.
- Recommend necessary support services for emotional, nutritional, financial and medical needs.
- Propose importance of follow-up-care not only for the patient but for family, friends, and sex partners.
- Prophylaxis may be recommended to persons of infected sex partners.
- Propose prophylactic therapy if HIV transmission is suspected, especially for sexual assault victims and abused children.

Your healthcare provider with consultation with experts (if need be), may propose a treatment option for your current condition. It's heart-wrenching that AIDS has no effective cure yet, but there have been some very promising advances in HIV/AIDS treatment and control. Life cycle of HIV offers some clues - key steps in this process can be blocked, changed, mimicked, or modified by medications such as protease inhibitors, non-nucleoside reverse transcriptase inhibitors (NNRTIs), and others as described in this chapter. Experienced and specialized healthcare providers in the U.S. and elsewhere provide advanced customized care to patients by dispensing combination therapy and counseling. Patients are periodically tested for various opportunistic infections and treated. CD4 cell count and viral load tests are administered at intervals to monitor patients' progress, current health status, and determine if other procedures are necessary. Ideal treatment plan will produce favorable results such as:

- Lower viral load.
- Improve immune stimulation.
- Increase CD4 cell count and enhance immune process resulting in fewer episodes of opportunistic infections.
- Overall improvement in health eventually can result in normal living.

Extensive ongoing research has introduced many new and innovative antiviral drugs to fight HIV/AIDS menace, opportunistic infections, and resulting cancers. Some such drugs are listed below.

## Antiviral Drugs:

New and innovative medications offer true hope for millions infected by HIV. These newer drugs administered individually or in combination (cocktail) have proven to prolong life expectancy of HIV/AIDS victims. Many HIV patients live longer with no onset of AIDS or complications. Deaths due to AIDS are delayed and in many cases prevented. Opportunistic infections and HIV induced diseases are also either prevented or managed with better outcome. This is the direct result of advances in medical research, improved treatment, professional counseling, and care. Groups of medications of miracle drugs listed below are currently available to treat and manage HIV.

Your healthcare provider may prescribe appropriate combination, dosage, sequence, and frequency of single or cocktail regimen(s) as per most current CDC treatment guidelines.

## Nucleoside and Nucleotide (NRTI & NtRTI) analogues:

This group of antiviral drugs is a welcome relief not only for HIV/AIDS patients but also to millions who may suffer from other painful and deadly viral infections. The analogues used as prescribed can disrupt life cycle of retrovirus thus preventing assembly and multiplication. Patients' unique condition, disease status, and many other complex factors determine the specific drug or multiple drug (cocktail) treatment. Drugs administered appropriately inhibit/block one or more critical genome sites or essential phase of HIV life cycle. Virus assembly process (multiplication) can no longer continue. A list of available analogues affecting specific phase is compiled below:

1. **Viral Entry Inhibitors or Fusion/ Attachment Inhibitors:**
   Interfere with binding and attachment of the virus to CD4 lymphocyte.
2. **Receptor Antagonist Analogues:**
   Prevent viral binding to CD4 cell wall as a result virus fail to enter CD4 cell.
3. **Integrase Inhibitors:**
   Prevent viral RNA integration with host DNA, a key phase in the assembly of virulent virus. The drug inhibits integrase activity.

**4. Nucleoside and Nucleotide Reverse Transcriptase Inhibitors (NRTIs & NtRTIs):**
Prevent viral DNA from reverting to infectious RNA.

**5. Non-nucleoside Reverse Transcriptase Inhibitors (NNRTI):**
Block the genetic attachment site thus prevent viral reverse transcription.

**6. Protease Inhibitors (PIs):**
Prevent virus assembly by inhibiting protease activity that is essential for final viral assembly.

**7. Maturation Inhibitors:**
Prevent virus maturation by blocking newly produced poly-protein into mature capsid protein (p24) of HIV. A defective virus may be non-virulent.

Most antiviral drugs developed to perform specific functions described above are administered individually or in cocktail regimens. However current recommended standard of HIV care is to administer cocktail approach or combination drug therapy. Cocktail may include one or two nucleoside analogues and one non-nucleoside analogue or a protease inhibitor (triple cocktail). Most pharmaceutical companies have recently introduced cocktail dosages to help and encourage combination therapy. Some such frequently prescribed cocktail combinations are listed below.

## FDA Approved Antiviral Drugs (Cocktail Combinations):

1. **Atripla:** Efavirenz, Emtricitabine, and Tenofovir (Triple cocktail)
2. **Combivir:** Lamivudine and Zidovudine

3. **Complera:** Emtricitabine, Rilpivirine, and Tenofovir (Triple cocktail)
4. **Epzicom (USA) or Kivexa (Europe):** Abacavir and Lamivudine
5. **Kaletra:** Lopinavir and Ritonavir
6. **Stribilor:** Cobicistat, Elvitetegravir, and Emtricitabine or Lenofovir (Triple cocktail)
7. **Trizivir:** Abacavir, Lamivudine, and Zudovudine (Triple cocktail)
8. **Truvada\*:** Emtricitabine and Tenofovir
   *FDA approved Tuvada in pill form is currently available for treatment. Please read Prognosis at the end of this chapter.

## Healthcare provider preferred combination drug therapy in the U.S.:

1. Emtricitabine and Tenofovir (2 NRTIs) and Efavirenz (NNRTI)
2. Emtricitabine, Tenofovir, and Raltegravir (Integrase Inhibitor)
3. Emtricitabine, Tenofovir, and Darunavir or Ritonavir (Protease Inhibitors)
4. Emtricitabine, Tenofovir, and Atazanavir or Ritonavir (Protease Inhibitors)

Most healthcare experts agree that antiviral therapy be initiated upon thorough evaluation and disease status of HIV/AIDS patient (s). Certain standard of care guidelines must be applied in order to select qualifying candidates. Once instituted, therapy must never be stopped. This approach is recommended in the greater health concern for the patient. In the absence of regular, scheduled administration of antiviral drugs, chances are more virulent strains may become predominant and drug resistant therefore increase fatalities in the long run. New strains can also present additional problems and worse yet, new infections.

HIV positive children and adolescents often experience rapid progression of the disease. Healthcare professionals therefore take great pains to provide much aggressive treatment and follow – up care to the youngsters. Most victims of sexual assault and physical abuse are provided post-exposure prophylaxis treatment (PEP) however PEP is not effective 72 hours post-exposure in most cases.

Most antiviral drugs have serious adverse effects especially among children and patients of advanced age. Healthcare providers and medical staff make every effort to inform and educate all patients who qualify for antiviral drug therapy. Some such adverse effects are listed below:

- Older patients and some children do not respond well to drug therapy.
- Many patients are intolerant to antiviral drugs.
- Patients usually develop resistance to drugs. However if a dose is missed for whatever reason greater drug resistance may be in the cards.
- Serious side effects such as chills, diarrhea, headache, lymph node swelling associated with pain, sore throat, weakness, and weight loss are common among patients with advanced disease.
- Lack of appetite, depression, and memory loss is also common.

- Some may experience persistent and recurring flu-like symptoms.
- Most patients who start drug therapy may continue to experience some symptoms as described already.

Almost all antiviral drugs come with a cost prohibitory price tag. Annual cost for drug therapy may exceed several thousand dollars per patient. Most patients especially victims from poor and under developed countries can hardly afford newer antiviral cocktail therapy. Several International organizations and charitable institutions are engaged in providing help and monetary support to such victims. Healthcare providers, local hospital, public library, local Red Cross, and media can assist people contact such organizations.

## Treatment and Management of Accidental Exposure to HIV:

Some people by virtue of their profession, sex, and age are at risk for HIV. The list below may not be complete but covers most such groups.

- Professionals such as healthcare providers, medical personnel, medical research staff, hospital staff, and nursing home staff.
- Personnel in charge of group homes, institutional living, dormitories, correctional facilities, and prisons.
- Victims of sexual assault.
- Victims of child abuse.
- Victims of aggression and physical violence.
- Commercial sex workers.

Some risk for HIV, hepatitis B, and C infections is a constant threat and a serious health hazard for all health-care providers and medical personnel all over the world. All healthcare providers in the U.S. receive education, training, and scheduled procedural updates on the job and even before they enter job market. U.S. department of Labor sponsored Occupational Safety & Health Administration (OSHA) guidelines are mandated by law in all states. The real risk of exposure, unintended severe consequences, and ways to avoid them are discussed in order to help preserve a healthy, risk-free work force. When accidents do happen and people are exposed to risk, appropriate treatment is made available with extreme urgency. In the U.S., employers must document all accidental exposures, secure blood samples for baseline testing, provide medical treatment, and counseling in the event of job-related incident(s). All such persons receive prophylactic treatment with antiretroviral drugs and closely monitored. Almost all such drugs have very unpleasant side effects therefore most recipients discontinue therapy before full course. However it's wise and medically prudent to complete the treatment as prescribed to avoid future health risks.

Elaborate comprehensive treatment plan is also available for other forms of high risk exposures such as sexual abuse/assault, and rape. All such victims also receive therapy, prophylactic treatment, and periodic blood tests for HIV antigen/antibody, hepatitis B, hepatitis C, and other STDs if indicated. Regular check-up and intense counseling is also made available.

All victims of rape and sexual abuse must be treated with great urgency - medical procedures and blood tests included. Only most reliable and accurate blood tests must be requested to avoid much emotional, mental, and psychological trauma to the already battered victim. This approach is expedient and legally/medically beneficial to all parties concerned.

Victims of aggression or violent crime are also at risk therefore need treatment and care as above.

HIV/AIDS patients are usually hospitalized upon medical assessment for treatment and care. Hospitals and clinics in the U.S. prefer not to isolate HIV positive patients unless they have contagious opportunistic infections such as tuberculosis. Persons exposed to accidental needle sticks, lacerations, and injury may be treated as out- patients.

Most healthcare providers and clinics in the U.S. recognize that most newly diagnosed HIV positive person needs expert professional counseling and care therefore recommend such services with great sense of compassion and urgency.

## Follow – Up Services:

Most primary healthcare providers expect trauma, distress, and helplessness not to mention anger and anguish among newly diagnosed HIV positive people. HIV positive persons face enormous obstacles, life changing adaptive challenges, physical, and emotional issues such as stress and anxiety. For many victims unforeseen events such as employment, relationships, family, and myriad other changes may be in the offing.

Newly diagnosed men, women, adolescents, and children require unique customized care for physical and emotional needs. In the U.S., most primary healthcare providers refer HIV positive persons to specialized professionals for follow – up services such as:

- Expert medical evaluation by physicians/clinics specializing in treatment and care of HIV patients.
- Behavioral and psychological evaluation by professionals.

Most cities and communities in the U.S. provide follow-up services with patient's unique situation in mind. The strategy is to design and execute a holistic approach to suit most urgent needs at hand. As the initial barriers are carefully overcome a more sustainable long term plan may be devised to include the following:

- Immediate and long term medical implications of HIV infection clearly explained so the patient is prepared for abrupt changes.
- Importance of medications, proper dosage, and frequency must be emphasised.
- Emotional support to cope with anger, depression, and other issues.
- Behavior changes, avoiding risk, and protecting friends and family are suggested.

Professional counseling can successfully accomplish general and specific goals of new and not so new HIV diagnosed people. Community based non-profit organizations in the U.S. actively participate and provide support for several great causes - HIV/AIDS is one such great cause. HIV positive people are encouraged to join local groups and caring organizations for counseling and support.

## Management of Sex and Needle Sharing Drug Partners:

Early detection and treatment of HIV can reduce pain, suffering, and death. Therefore patients' sex/needle sharing partners must be identified and treated with great urgency. Healthcare providers must ensure that patients comply. Partners can be identified and notified confidentially by:

- Patient referrals – Patients directly inform sex or needle sharing partners about their HIV positive status and suggest seek help ASAP.
- Provider referral – Trained healthcare professionals locate sex and needle sharing partners based on patient information. They are informed of increased risk for HIV and offered confidential consultation and testing.
- Partners who were exposed to HIV patient (s) within the preceding 72 hours should be offered post-exposure prophylaxis.

New patients and recently identified sex/needle sharing partners require follow-up care as described above and treatment if indicated.

## Prevention of HIV/AIDS:

Your goal must be to develop and implement effective strategies that work best for you. Local hospitals, community organizations, religious, and non-profit groups in the U.S. provide educational programs and support services to all interested persons. Community leaders, educators, religious affiliates, and social activists in many communities also help promote awareness, dangers of risky behavior(s), and overall understanding of AIDS. The righteous controversies aside, lives we save may well worth the rewards. In the U.S. most states and concerned communities provide education and actively encourage persons of high risk use preventive tools such as condoms and clean needles. Better yet, many communities distribute these devices free of charge. Public awareness about this life-threatening disease will save lives and spare human suffering in the long run therefore even greater effort must be made to inform and counsel all sexually active adults, alcoholics, drug users, and persons at high risk about the imminent dangers and harsh consequences of reckless behavior.

The message emphasizing benefits of prevention with the alternative of nuclear option of treatment (with unpleasant side-effects) may sink in if delivered to a receptive age group – it is worth the effort. Strategy to prevent HIV/AIDS can be implemented by following a multi-prong approach as described below.

## 1. Uninfected healthy adults and teens:

- Prevention of HIV can be accomplished to some degree by identifying the age group(s) at greatest risk. Sex education with emphasis on abstinence may get some attention from teens and adults.

- Risky sexual behaviors must be pointed out, alternate safe sex practices recommended, and health benefits emphacised.
- Safe sex prevents HIV and other common STDs.
- Surest way to prevent HIV or any other STD is abstain from sex altogether or have sex with only with someone who is NOT infected (have it confirmed) and has sex ONLY with you.

## 2. HIV positive people:

- Most preferred practice is greater emphasis on abstinence that will eliminate risk to others.
- Safe and protected sex is also critically important. It's risk free. Barrier to blood and body fluid transfer may decrease risk but not completely.
- Prospective sex partner(s) must be informed about your HIV positive status so he/she can avoid infection.
- Antiretroviral therapy may halt progression of HIV but not transmission of virus to sex partners.
- Sex partners of HIV positive patients can avoid infection by antiretroviral suppressive therapy – consult your physician.
- Transmission of HIV from infected mothers to infants can be prevented by drug therapy during pregnancy. Consider discussing this option with your physician.

- HIV positive mothers run the risk of transmitting HIV through breast milk – though such risk is low, it is still a risk. In many poor underdeveloped countries an alternative is not available. In the U. S. and many developed countries where clean water and quality infant food and formulas are readily available, mothers must consider this alternative and abstain from breast feeding.
- HIV positive childbearing age women must consult their healthcare providers before getting pregnant. Impending risk and potential infection to the baby must be avoided.
- Your physician may recommend avoiding pregnancy if that is an option for you. Accept such medical advice gracefully and discuss alternatives.
- If and when you learn about your HIV positive status, promptly notify (directly or through your healthcare provider) all previous and current sex/needle share partners - it's compassionate. Timely intervention and prompt medical help may save much suffering and even lives.

### 3. Alcoholics and drug abusers:
Alcoholics and drug users must recognize that they have a problem. If unable to quit on your own, consider joining support groups such as Alcoholics Anonymous and Drug Treatment (rehab) program.

Alcoholics and druggies in most situations don't make the right choices because their decision making ability is impaired.

- Reusing/sharing needle MUST STOP. You and your accomplice are at much higher risk for HIV, hepatitis B, and C when contaminated needles are used repeatedly.
- Free condoms and clean needles may be available in your community. Local health department, STD clinic, and your healthcare provider can assist – just inquire.

## 4. Dental and medical staff:

- Make yourself familiar with OSHA guidelines – used needles, medical waste, blood, body fluids, tissue, urine, stool, and other contaminated objects must be handled as per OSHA guidelines.
- Whenever there is probability of contact with patients, elderly, medical waste (as described above), and other soiled objects routinely wear latex gloves. If you are allergic to latex find safe gloves made of other material.
- Be alert at all times. Do not expose your patients nor be exposed to any risk. Your desire to help patients and save lives should be risk free at all times. Your good health will save more lives in the long run.
- Healthcare professionals need to be familiar with face masks, gloves, and universal precautions.

The strategy of compassionate communication can result in greater caring and real support for victims. Social stigma will eventually disappear as the beneficial message and mantra of power of prevention start producing results. As more and more people understand AIDS, discrimination will also end for patients who are unjustly denied housing, jobs, medical care, and health insurance. In the U.S., federal government and several states have enacted laws to protect AIDS patients. Some states have also streamlined laws to protect confidentiality of medical records related to HIV/AIDS. Punishing victims of AIDS on presumed guilty (wrong) grounds or any premise by denying medical care and dignified living is immoral, unjustified, and counterproductive. Following useful tips are for healthcare providers, educators, community/religious leaders, and social activists.

- Promote awareness about all facets of HIV/ AIDS such as risks, transmission, infection, symptoms, and treatment.
- Provide education to adults and teens on topics such as safe sex, methods/techniques for STDs prevention, and expected healthy/safe behavior. Mythical risky behaviors must be corrected.
- Sex Education through presentation of facts should not be construed as promoting promiscuity.
- Discuss the benefits of pre-exposure and post-exposure prophylaxis.
- Discrimination prevention will encourage HIV/ AIDS victims to seek and receive prompt professional care.

- Promote harmony and cooperation. Avoid controversy and blame game so AIDS victims feel safe and free of stigma. Encourage patients to seek professional help, counseling, guidance, and support.

## Prognosis:

Medical research is underway to develop effective vaccines for HIV. Though there is much progress, at present such vaccines are not available for immunization.

Several drug combination and cocktail injectable therapies are currently available to suppress rapid HIV progression. Patient's current disease status usually dictates the best combination or cocktail.

FDA has recently introduced Truvada (Emtricitabine and Tenofovir) pill that has value and promise to millions infected by HIV. Truvada inhibits activity of viral protein that attack CD4 cells to initiate HIV infection. Truvada pill can suppress new infections and prevent reinfections. Therefore can be an effective prophylactic medication for suppressive therapy. Talk to your liver specialist if Truvada is good for you. Truvada can provide benefits such as:

- Suppress and reduce risk for HIV infection and reinfection.
- Benefit victims of sexual assault and abuse as a therapeutic regimen.
- Can be prescribed to persons for post-exposure and pre-exposure episodes.
- Truvada is recommended for heterosexual HIV negative partner (s) whose partner has HIV.

Risk can be reduced if both take Truvada as directed by specialists.

- Truvada is also recommended for MSM HIV negative men who may have multiple sex partners of unknown etiology.
- Truvada pill must be taken as directed by your healthcare giver for best results.

## Other Benefit Truvada pills provide Include:

- Pills can be taken as prescribed by mouth in the privacy of home – no painful, prolonged intravenous procedure.
- Patients save time, money, and inconvenience of travel to distant clinics or medical facilities.

## However Truvada does not:

- Cure HIV.
- Prevent HIV transmission from a positive person to sex partners.
- Prevent opportunistic infections among HIV persons.

# HIV/AIDS - Opportunistic Infections - Co - Infections

Victims of HIV/AIDS are at great risk for acquiring several opportunistic infections (OIs). This is mainly due to their compromised immune status - CD4 lymphocyte cell count being low and viral load too high. Ironically, a vast majority of deaths associated with HIV/AIDS are due to recurring co- infections or OIs. A brief description of such deadly opportunistic infections is provided below.

## A. Tuberculosis -TB
## Mycobacterium tuberculosis

Tuberculosis, an acutely contagious airborne disease kills approximately 1.7 million people world-wide each year. TB, the most common opportunistic infection among HIV/ AIDS patients is often fatal. Someone acquires TB every few seconds.

Mycobacterium tuberculosis usually infects lungs but can infect any part of the body such as abdominal cavity, bladder, brain, joints, kidney, reproductive organs, pericardium, and spine.

TB is very common in most poor third world countries yet no stranger to the affluent western world.

Antibiotics such as streptomycin (1940s), isoniazid (1950s), ethambutol (1960s), and rifampin (1970s) managed to contain tuberculosis to some extent. In the 1980s AIDS epidemic combined with conditions such as overcrowding, poor hygiene, increasing prison population, slums, and homeless shelters contributed heavily to the rise of TB. Emergence of antibiotic resistant tubercle strains also compounded already existing serious health care crisis.

In most countries, TB is the leading cause of death among HIV/AIDS patients. Impaired immune system of an HIV infected person provides Mycobacterium a perfect opportunity to jumpstart, attack, and infect. For most HIV/AIDS patients risk of reactivation of latent TB is also very high.

## Transmission of Tuberculosis:

People inhale airborne microbes when in close proximity to infected persons and develop active or inactive (latent) TB. Active TB -is a serious condition. An active TB patient is highly contagious and can spread the germs by coughing, sneezing, and spitting. Inactive or latent TB is "contained" by the immune system therefore people with latent TB are not ill, have no symptoms, and non - contagious. This condition may last a life time for some people. But for HIV/ AIDS patients latent TB can quickly become active.

Pregnant women can infect the baby before or during childbirth.

This Guide deals with active TB of the lungs especially among HIV/AIDS patients.

## Symptoms:

Symptoms usually appear within a few days after exposure.

- Chills, fever, and night sweat.
- Fatigue, weakness, and fainting spell.
- Progressive weight loss.
- Most patients infected with TB also have persistent productive cough usually mixed with blood.
- Persistent acute chest pain and shortness of breath.

## Diagnosis:

Pulmonary TB is presumptively diagnosed by patient's symptoms. Skin test, acid fast stain test of sputum, and sputum culture must be requested to confirm initial diagnosis. Skin test may be misleading among HIV/AIDS patients therefore laboratory results of acid fast test and sputum culture is critical. Chest x-ray is also made to confirm diagnosis and extent of lung damage.

Tuberculosis, active or latent presents a herculean challenge to the medical community due to in great part the HIV/AIDS epidemic. Recently diagnosed as well as existing HIV patients are at much higher risk of acquiring active tuberculosis. HIV positive persons with a history of latent tuberculosis are at much greater risk of reactivation. This alarming trend is real - the risk is real - therefore preventive strategies must be devised to counter situations such as:

- Increase in active tuberculosis worldwide.
- Increase in latent tuberculosis worldwide.
- Increase of tuberculosis infection transmission worldwide.
- More HIV patients infected with tuberculosis worldwide.

In the U.S., above trend has adversely affected already deteriorating health care crisis. Supportive mechanism and resources are already stretched to the limit.

Among most poor nations and third world countries where HIV/TB epidemic is rapidly getting out of control, situation is much worse. A shrinking world, easy access to all parts of the globe by air, sea, and land has greatly increased the risk of TB, especially among HIV positive and even HIV negative people. The ease of transmission of TB also complicates already worsening situation.

- TB is easily spread (aerosol) and harder to diagnose in HIV infected persons.

- Many unsuspecting new episodes result in more infections.
- Tuberculosis can be fatal to HIV infected people - much more serious than any other opportunistic infection.

## Treatment:

Tuberculosis infection for most HIV/AIDS patients can be fatal if not treated aggressively. Hospitalized patients are usually isolated. Simultaneous treatment for HIV and TB is a unique medical challenge for healthcare givers worldwide. Only effective antibiotics to cure TB and promising antiviral drugs are used to avoid treatment failure and complications.

Most healthcare providers in the U.S. and elsewhere can professionally treat and manage this highly complex health problem with modern technological advances and newer antibiotics. Treatment for TB can differ for patients depending upon their unique situation (s). Prompt treatment also prevents active transmission of bacteria. Customized care and treatment for HIV with preferred cocktail therapy must be instituted for favorable outcome.

Tuberculosis can be prevented to some extent by mass vaccination but the efficacy of BCG (Bacille Calmette-Guerin) vaccine is questionable. Therefore, a more effective and reliable vaccine needs to be developed for mass vaccination. Preventive drug therapy namely isoniazid (INH) is recommended to high risk people and those with latent tuberculosis. The world health organization (WHO) also recommends this approach for HIV positive population with latent TB.

## B. Pneumocystis pneumonia- PCP
## Pneumocystis Jiroveci (formerly P. carinii)

Pneumocystis jiroveci bacterium is a normal lung flora. The organism is non-pathogenic, causes no disease, nor discomfort among healthy people. But when body's defenses are compromised because of cancer, chemotherapy, and HIV/AIDS the organism can cause lung infection. In the early stages of AIDS epidemic, recurring Pneumocystis jiroveci pneumonia (PCP) was a major concern for AIDS victims. More than 80 percent of AIDS patients who don't receive standard prophylactic care develop PCP at some stage of HIV/AIDS. Effective preventive medications and greater awareness have significantly reduced incidence of PCP. In most AIDS patients PCP causes severe lung infection, respiratory disease, and even death. Even though death rate has been drastically reduced with prompt treatment and care, PCP is still a credible threat for AIDS victims worldwide. For most HIV patients PCP is self- inflicted due to poor immune response.

## Symptoms:
Symptoms for PCP usually appear several weeks after onset of infection. Most common symptoms are:

- Fever and night sweat.
- Dry non-productive cough, shortness of breath, and breathing difficulties.
- Persistent acute chest pain.
- Weakness, depression, and lack of appetite.
- Progressive weight loss.

## Diagnosis:

Diagnosis is made by direct microscopic examination of first morning sputum specimen. If unable to detect microbes on slide, sputum culture for PCP is requested. Sputum can be obtained by inducing cough or bronchoscopy. Patient's HIV status, medical history, and recent sex partners who are also HIV positive are factors that help diagnose and confirm PCP.

## Treatment:

Recent advances in preventive management therapy and antiretroviral drugs have significantly reduced incidence of PCP in the U.S. Antibiotics are also prescribed to prevent PCP infection (prophylactic) altogether. Active PCP is aggressively treated with one or more antibiotics. Antibiotics are taken orally while aerosol dosage is delivered via respiratory tract directly to the lungs. This dual treatment approach has greater benefits not to mention fewer side effects. AIDS patients may have to continue antibiotic treatment for an indefinite period to prevent recurrence of PCP.

## C. Bacillary Angiomatosis - Cat-Scratch Disease
### Bartonella henselae

Bacillary angiomatosis, also known as cat-scratch disease is an infection caused by Bartonella henselae. Healthy people with no health issues normally heal cat scratch within 2 – 6 months. Immune challenged persons by contrast can develop infection at the site of cat scratch. Infection may become painful, severe, and systemic in persons with AIDS.

Most healthy cats are carriers of Bartonella henselae. Cats may playfully scratch pet owners to transmit microbes. Bartonella quintana, yet another related bacillus was the cause of trench fever among soldiers during World War I. Bartonella quintana is transmitted by body lice. In both cases the exposure will bring on bacillary angiomatosis, a severe infection of the blood vessels. This systemic infection can cause lesions similar to those for Kaposi sarcoma. Lesions or blisters may appear on the skin, mucosal lining, and organs such as liver and spleen.

## Symptoms:

Symptoms usually develop at the scratch site within 3-10 days after cat scratch that was totally ignored as nothing to worry. Symptoms may be much severe for elderly and HIV patients.

- Clusters of tiny pink/purple/red spots and blisters appear just under the skin. Blisters may be crusted, some containing pus (pustules).
- The lymph nodes (nodules) around the scratch area swell and become firm but tender for touch, bleed profusely if ruptured due to scratch, pressure, or puncture. If left alone nodules may fill with pus and drain through ruptured skin.
- HIV patients may experience severe pain as blisters spread and become systemic.
- Patient may develop fever, chills, headache, and sweats.
- Lack of appetite, nausea, and vomiting may follow.

- Some people may develop eye problems and in rare cases swelling of brain cells causing chronic headache.
- Almost all infected people with no underlying cause usually heal within 2-6 months.
- People with AIDS, cancers, and other malignancies may develop severe form of cat-scratch disease. Blood vessels may grow out of control and form large tumor-like masses in organs such as bone, lymph nodes, heart, liver, spleen, lungs, intestine, and respiratory tract.
- Persons receiving chemotherapy and medications for complex health issues can develop severe form of bacillary angiomatosis.
- Impaired breathing and blood circulation can be life threatening. Prompt diagnosis and treatment can save lives.

## Diagnosis:

Your healthcare provider must be informed about the cat-scratch. He/she can confirm diagnosis by the appearance of swollen lymph nodes. If not sure of a cat scratch blood test may confirm Bartonella henselae antibodies for diagnosis.

## Treatment:

Bacillary angiomatosis is effectively treated with antibiotics. Erythromycin is the antibiotic of choice, but several other antibiotics are also available for people who may be allergic or resistant to erythromycin.

Patients with life threatening ailments such as AIDS, cancers, and malignancies require more aggressive and prolonged antibiotic therapy. Patients are also hydrated, medications prescribed for pain, and pus drained from pustules and infected lymph nodes.

## D. Toxoplasmosis
## Toxoplasma gondii

Toxoplasmosis is an infection caused by Toxoplasma gondii, a single celled parasite. Toxoplasma is found in more than 80 % of all adults all over the world, causes no known episodes or ailment, yet may infect and cause distress of the central nervous system among AIDS patients. People with impaired immune system (CD4 cell count less than100) may also be affected. Pregnant women can transmit Toxoplasma to the fetus resulting in congenital toxoplasmosis, miscarriage, and stillbirth.

Cats are carriers of Toxoplasma gondii. Parasite produces eggs (oocytes) in the cats' intestinal lining that are shed with feces. People exposed to soil containing oocytes can get infected. Consuming raw or undercooked meat and meat products can also cause toxoplasma infection.

### Symptoms and disorders:
Toxoplasmosis can be mild or acute. Symptoms for mild and acute forms of Toxoplasmosis are described below.

## 1. Lymphatic (mild) toxoplasmosis:

- Slightly enlarged painless lymph nodes in the arm pits and neck.
- Mild fever that may last for weeks but resolves eventually.
- Muscle pain and feeling of illness.

- Disorders such as low blood pressure, low white cell count, and increased lymphocyte count (resembling infectious mononucleosis) is common.

## 2. Acute disseminated toxoplasmosis:
People with impaired immune system and victims of HIV/AIDS often develop acute toxoplasmosis. Common symptoms are:

- Flu-like symptoms such as high fever, chills, night sweats, and fatigue.
- Inflammation of brain, heart, liver, and lungs may lead to additional health problems such as meningo-encephalitis, myocarditis, hepatitis, and pneumonia.
- Inflammation of eyes may cause blurred vision and blindness.
- Convulsions leading to coma, confusion, diminished sensation, and headache.
- Lack of appetite, exhaustion, and rapid weight loss.
- Symptoms for children born with congenital toxoplasmosis may be severe and even fatal.

Toxoplasmosis in persons with HIV/AIDS can spread to organs such as brain, heart, liver, and lungs. Infection of the brain may result in brain inflammation (Meningo-encephalitis), diminished sensation, and paralysis. Severe brain infection may cause chronic headache, confusion, convulsions, trembling, coma, and even death. Heart, liver, and lung infection can be severe and even fatal for some.

## Diagnosis:

Toxoplasmosis can be diagnosed by antibody test. Patient history and symptoms may be helpful for accurate diagnosis. Pet cat (s) may also confirm suspicion along with blood test results. It is critically important that your doctor is informed if you suspect HIV or other STDs.

Persons with impaired immune system may require additional sophisticated diagnostic tests such as Magnetic Resonance Imaging (MRI) to determine damage to brain, eyes, heart, liver, and lungs.

## Treatment:

Your healthcare providers may prescribe medication (s) keeping your actual current health status in mind. People with HIV/AIDS usually experience frequent recurrence of toxoplasmosis therefore may receive prolonged or indefinite treatment to avoid recurrence and even death. Pregnant women are treated only if vital organs such as brain, eyes, or heart are infected.

## Prevention - Helpful Tips for HIV/AIDS Patients:

Prevention of toxoplasmosis is important for victims of AIDS. Toxoplasmosis in immune impaired individuals is often fatal. Following suggestions must be taken seriously to avoid unpleasant episodes of toxoplasmosis.

- Thoroughly wash hands often before and after handling food and pets.
- Avoid contact with cats while preparing/cooking food, and snacks.
- Avoid contact with cats during snacks, dinner, and desert.

- Thoroughly wash and rinse fruits and fresh vegetables.
- Cook all meat, poultry, and meat products well. Check temperature for safety with a food thermometer.
- Use heated then cooled (warm) plates and dishes to serve food at all times.
- Cat litter box must be handled with extreme care. Designate a healthy person to handle this chore. If you have no choice, wear disposable vinyl gloves and mask.
- Wash hands with soap and water soon after meals, care of your cat, and garden chores.

Prognosis for people who acquire toxoplasmosis with no underlying syndromes such as HIV/AIDS and malignancies is good however for immune impaired persons it can be often fatal if not promptly diagnosed and treated.

## E. Mycobacterium avium Complex Infection - MAC Mycobacterium avium and Mycobacterium intracellular

Mycobacterium avium and Mycobacterium intracellular, the two related bacteria cause Mycobacterium avium complex or MAC disease. This is one of the most common opportunistic infections among 35 – 45% of persons living with AIDS. Bacteria usually infect lungs but may also attack bones, lymph nodes, skin, and other organs. Middle aged people whose lungs have been weakened by bronchitis, emphysema, prolonged smoking, and latent TB are at higher risk.

MAC is often detected in people who suffer from AIDS for more than 2 years. Most AIDS patients infected by MAC have low CD4 cell count (less than 50) and also suffer from at least yet another opportunistic infection.

Mycobacteria (MAC complex) are normal habitats of nature and normally found in soil, water, dust, bird droppings, and animal feces. Most healthy people harbor MAC in their stomach and lungs with no episodes, symptoms, or infection. Immune compromised HIV/AIDS victims however are at high risk. Bacteria attack the lining of stomach wall and lungs. Once membranes are penetrated bacteria can enter the blood stream and spread to other parts of the body causing disseminated infection (septicemia). Mycobacteria are resistant to most common antibiotics, including those used to treat and contain tuberculosis.

MAC resembles/mimics tuberculosis but MAC is not contagious.

## Symptoms:
MAC disease causes symptoms similar to tuberculosis. Infection usually develops slowly among HIV/AIDS patients. Most symptoms include:

- Persistent cough with bloody mucus.
- Breathing trouble and shortness of breath.
- Chills, mild fever, headache, and dizzy spells.
- Fatigue, weight loss, restlessness, and lingering diarrhea.
- Low grade chest and abdominal pain.
- Slightly tender, swollen lymph nodes.
- Anemia and blood disorders.

## Diagnosis:

Chest x-ray can detect lung infection. Sputum culture is usually performed to grow and identify MAC and rule out tuberculosis. Sterile site samples such as blood, bone marrow, and cerebral/spinal fluid are also cultured to confirm MAC infection among HIV positive persons.

## Treatment:

MAC microbes are highly resistant to most antibiotics. Recent advances and newer antibiotics can check and delay progression of MAC infection. Improved immune system with elevated CD4 count is yet another option to delay rapid progress of MAC disease. Currently there is more hope than despair.

## Prevention – Helpful Tips for HIV/AIDS Patients:

Prevention of MAC is critically important to save lives. Following useful health-care tips can help prevent episodes of MAC and OIs among victims of HIV/AIDS and health conscious public. As pointed out already, it is difficult to avoid MAC microbes but with sustained effort and greater awareness risk and risky situations can be avoided.

- Always drink boiled water. MAC microbes can be found in most water systems including hospital water supply and bottled water.
- Avoid raw food and vegetables. Vegetables and salads from street vendors must be thoroughly washed and rinsed before consumption.
- Thoroughly wash and rinse fruits and vegetables. Peel fruits, tubers, and items for salads, desert, or just to eat.

- Tubers such beets, carrots, potatoes and sweet potatoes must be thoroughly washed, peeled, and rinsed before use.
- Avoid non-pasteurized milk and cheese.
- Avoid physical contact with birds and animals. Bird droppings (even pet birds) may contain MAC microbes. Pigeons, common in most cities can transmit Cryptococcus an opportunistic infectious agent to persons with HIV.
- Excessive and even moderate alcohol consumption must be avoided. Alcoholic AIDS patients are highly susceptible to MAC disease.

## F. Histoplasmosis
### Fungal Infection
### Histoplasma capsulatum

Fungus Histoplasma capsulatum causes histoplasmosis, an infection of the lungs. Anyone can get this disease but usually most long-term smokers, TB patients, and HIV/AIDS victims are at much higher risk. HIV positive people are more likely to develop severe form of histoplasmosis. Besides lungs, the infection can spread to liver, spleen, lymph nodes, intestine, mouth, and other organs of the body.

Histoplasma grows in soil that's contaminated with bat and bird droppings. Fungus produces powdery spores that can become airborne. Heavy inhalation of spores can cause serious respiratory infection among farmers and gardeners.

Histoplasmosis is a cause of concern all over the world, but it is prevalent in river valleys and tropics. In the United States, it is most common in the Mississippi, Ohio, and river valleys of the East.

## Symptoms:

Most people who are infected by histoplasmosis are asymptomatic. Those who get infected as described above may develop symptoms for acute, chronic, and progressive form of histoplasmosis.

   **1. Acute:** In acute form of the disease symptoms may appear 3 – 21 days post exposure to fungal spores. Resulting lung infection may cause symptoms such as:

- Chest pain, mild fever, and feeling of illness (malaise).
- Dry non-productive cough generally appears within 1- 2 weeks after exposure.
- Increased breathing difficulty.
- In most healthy people these mild symptoms usually disappear without treatment within 2 – 6 weeks.

   **2. Chronic:** Chronic cavitary form of lung infection develops gradually. Symptoms appear several weeks post-exposure. Most symptoms listed below may be much severe than for acute form of histoplasmosis.

- Chest pain, mild fever, and a feeling of illness (malaise).
- Lack of appetite and weight loss.
- Breathing difficulty associated with intense cough. Some people may cough large amounts of blood resulting in severe lung damage and even death.

- Most healthy people recover without treatment within 2-6 months but most HIV victims require treatment and care to resolve cough, prevent damage to lungs and scarring of organs.

**3. Progressive:** Disseminated form of histoplasmosis usually affects immune impaired persons, especially HIV/AIDS patients. People receiving chemotherapy for various forms of cancers and malignancies are also at great risk. Most symptoms listed above normally appear but much severe. Symptoms may worsen gradually or abruptly. Such symptoms for progressive form of histoplasmosis are listed below.

- Liver, lymph nodes, and spleen may enlarge due to swelling.
- Infection may also cause blisters or ulcers in the mouth and stomach.
- In some severe cases adrenal glands may be infected resulting in Addison's disease.
- If untreated, infection can be fatal for most immune impaired people.
- Aggressive treatment can prevent fatalities among AIDS patients. Immune impaired persons require long term treatment, periodic follow-up and skilled care.
- Without treatment this form of histoplasmosis is fatal for >90% patients. Death may occur abruptly.

## Diagnosis:

Most severe infections are found among immune impaired people such as HIV/AIDS, leukemia, recent transplant recipients, and corticosteroid therapy dependents. Appropriate samples such as blood, sputum, and urine may be required for culture and identification of histoplasma. Ulcers in the mouth may be swabbed for culture. In rare cases needle aspiration from infected lymph nodes or a liver biopsy may be performed.

## Treatment:

Healthy people resolve acute histoplasmosis within 2-6 weeks with no treatment. Some people may feel sick temporarily but symptoms quickly disappear. Rarely healthy people require antifungal medications to overcome breathing difficulty.

Most people with chronic cavitary form of the disease recover without treatment within few months. Breathing problems may continue and may worsen for some requiring aggressive treatment. Untreated patients may cough up large amounts of blood causing severe lung damage and in rare cases even death.

Progressive histoplasmosis affects only immune impaired people. Symptoms may aggravate gradually or worsen abruptly as several organs may be affected. Most patients respond to aggressive intravenous/oral treatment but without prompt treatment disease can be fatal. Some AIDS patients may die even with treatment. Recent advances in skillful management and care of histoplasmosis (such as those with AIDS, cancers, and malignancies) has saved many lives.

## Prevention:

Histoplasmosis can be prevented by limiting exposure to fungal spores. Immune compromised persons need to follow steps listed below:

- Avoid landscapes frequented by birds and bats such as farms, forests, and parks.
- Avoid exposure to dust, soil, and manure dumps.
- If you must be out or working in areas heavy with bird/bat traffic choose disposable clothing and a face mask.
- Hot/cold shower with generous soap and water post outing is very helpful in minimizing risk.
- Make yourself familiar with geographical areas with high density of histoplasma spores, such as bird sanctuaries, farms, forests, parks, tropics, valleys, and river basin (s) - avoid them if possible.

## G. Herpes
## Oral and Genital herpes
## Herpes simplex 1 & 2

Herpes simplex virus (HSV) causes chronic life-long infection of the skin and the mucous membrane. Recurring eruption/infection produces small, painful, fluid filled blisters. Repeat outbreak of herpes is frequent among 70-80 % people with HIV. Recurring prodromes are usually severe, intensely painful, and long lasting. Even as infection subsides, virus remains dormant inside the ganglia (nerve cells) that provide sensory nerves to affected areas such as genitals and the mouth. Periodically the dormant virus is reactivated by certain drugs, food, and some unknown factors. Prodrome may also be triggered by fever, overexposure to sunlight, stress, and waste syndrome. Persons with HIV and HSV are highly infectious during frequent outbreaks of HSV.

## Two types of viruses cause infection:

1. HSV-1: Causes infection of the mouth and lips – cold sores.
2. HSV-2: Causes anogenital infection.

## Transmission:

- Herpes I and 2 are transmitted by physical contact, body fluid exchange, and sexual intercourse.
- Virus can be transmitted when susceptible individuals come into direct contact with oral or genital blisters.
- Saliva and genital secretions of infected people contain high concentration of virus especially during herpes outbreak.
- Victims of sexual assault and abuse are at high risk.

## Symptoms:

General symptoms for herpes I and 2 are listed under Herpes Virus Infection (# 4 in this section). Most symptoms described here apply to people with HIV/AIDS. Patient's HIV status and degree of immune deficiency may aggravate symptoms.

- Feeling of discomfort, itching, and tingling preceded by classical herpes blisters either on the genitals, mouth, and anorectal area.
- Recurring herpes infections are particularly severe and extremely painful.
- Inflammation of the esophagus and intestine is common.
- Nerve abnormalities around the areas of repeated outbreak such as ano/genitals and oral.
- Patients with severe form of the disease can also acquire pneumonia, hepatitis, and complications of the central nervous system.

## Diagnosis:

Location of the blisters in the genital or oral region is very helpful in the diagnosis of herpes I and 2 as described under Herpes Viral Infection in this section. Detailed diagnostic procedures are also discussed in that section.

## Treatment:

People with AIDS and conditions where impaired immunity is a factor recurring herpes outbreak can be very severe and extremely painful. Experienced specialist must be consulted for much skilled care. Most people infected by only herpes I and 2 heal with treatment options listed below:

- Cleaning blisters with antiseptic soap and water.
- Keeping the infected area dry. Moist environment may cause bacterial/fungal infection.

- Antibacterial and antifungal creams prevent infections. Antiviral creams help heal blisters if placed directly on the blisters/ulcers/sores.
- Suppressive therapy for recurrent genital/oral herpes offers relief to millions by reducing frequency of symptomatic outbreaks hence fewer new infections.
- People who suffer from AIDS and impaired immune system must be referred to specialist(s) for state of the art skilled care.

## Prevention: How to lower risk for herpes?

Genital and oral herpes infections are difficult to prevent but efforts must be made to lower risk:

- Many infected people are asymptomatic and not aware of their infection.
- Most such people have mild suspicious symptoms when prodromes do occur. Virus culture, PCR, and type specific serology tests performed before and after prodromes can provide useful diagnostic information.
- Condoms used as indicated can reduce risk but condom protects only the area that covers - the penis. Other parts of the body such as lower abdomen, groin, and genitals are prone to herpes.
- Abstinence during prodromes may be very helpful. However surest way a person can prevent herpes is total abstinence. Or have sex only with a uninfected person who is monogamous.

- Contrary to street talk washing, urinating, or douching after sex neither prevents herpes nor reduces risk.

For more detailed information please refer to chapter # 4 of this section under Herpes Virus Infection.

## H. Hepatitis C
## Hepatitis C Virus – HCV

Hepatitis C is the most common blood borne infection in the United States. Currently over 3.2 million Americans are known to be chronically infected. About 20-30 percent of HIV infected people in the U.S. also acquire hepatitis C as an opportunistic infection. For most HIV infected persons dreaded destruction of the liver by HCV progresses much more rapidly, causes severe irreversible damage, and eventual death. HCV co-infection related hospital admissions in the United States are on the rise so are fatalities. Caring for HIV patients with HCV is also a shared concern among healthcare providers. These patients need added support (emotional, psychological, and medical) and much skilled care. Management of HCV and HIV, a complex combination is a huge medical challenge worldwide.

## Transmission:

- Infected person can transmit the disease to sex partners.
- Saliva and body fluids such as blood, genital secretions, and wound exudate can transmit HCV.

- Needle sharing drug users are at much greater risk for HCV.
- Recipients of blood and blood products were at considerable risk but at present most such products are screened for hepatitis C virus.
- Victims of sexual assault, rape, and abuse are at much greater risk. Most predators may be infected.
- Persons having tattoos done in places of questionable integrity are at risk.

## Symptoms:

Most HCV infected and newly infected persons can be asymptomatic - many for life. Some may experience mild transient symptoms. As symptoms go away, so does the anxiety and reason to seek medical help.

Most symptoms for hepatitis C are listed under Hepatitis C Viral Infections in this section. Some of the symptoms listed below are common for HIV positive people with chronic hepatitis C co-infection.

- Mild fever, feeling of illness, lack of appetite, and fatigue.
- Off and on upper abdominal pain due to inflammation of the liver.
- Jaundice, nausea, and vomiting.
- Disease may rapidly escalate for HIV/AIDS victims causing liver failure and certain death.
- HIV/AIDS victims usually experience much rapid progression of symptoms.

## Diagnosis:

A definitive diagnosis for hepatitis C can be made with patients' medical history, prevailing symptoms, and liver function tests. Blood test can also detect HCV RNA within 2-4 weeks of exposure and antibodies within 8-10 weeks. However liver biopsy may be required to determine severity of inflammation and degree of cirrhosis (destruction of liver tissue).

## Treatment:

People with HCV live for years with no symptoms and no liver damage. But for those with HIV/AIDS living with HCV can be a nightmare. Therefore it is critically important that prompt medical and supportive care be received. Patient(s) must consult an engaging healthcare provider such as a liver specialist who is familiar with recent technological advances and treatment options. Highly active antiviral therapy (HAART) combined with several precautionary preventive measures to suppress opportunistic infections are recommended to persons living with HIV/HCV.

## Prevention:

An effective vaccine for hepatitis C is not available yet. Post exposure prophylactic treatment with immunoglobulin is too ineffective. Prevention of HCV therefore requires practical methods such as:

- Reduce HCV transmission by promoting awareness among people at greater risk. Serious nature of HCV infection, chronic liver disease (CLD), and even death should be impressed upon through education.

- Effective preventive methods should be suggested to people at high risk such as persons sharing needles for drug use, and sex partners.
- Barrier methods and pre-exposure options should be encouraged.
- HCV infected people must be identified, counseled, and treated if indicated in order to prevent CLD and other debilitating syndromes.

People with HIV/HCV must be extremely careful and selective in choosing partners for sex and pleasure. Persons with HIV/HCV are at much higher risk to acquire other dreadful STDs and disorders therefore must painstakingly avoid risks.

## I. Cryptosporidiosis
## Cryptosporidium parvum

Cryptosporidiosis is a serious emerging opportunistic infection caused by an intestinal parasite, cryptosporidium. Parasite can cause gastroenteritis among persons with impaired immune response but not among healthy. Diarrhea caused by bacteria, drugs, food, and parasites is only an inconvenience to healthy people but can be fatal to persons with HIV/AIDS. Most elderly and infants are also at risk for gastroenteritis caused by cryptosporidium.

Cryptosporidium is usually found in feces of humans and animals. Cryptosporidium cysts, the oocytes can be present in food, soil, and water. Ingesting contaminated food and water can cause infection. 5,304 cryptosporidiosis episodes were reported in the U.S. in 2010.

## Symptoms:

Healthy individuals may have mild symptoms but symptoms among HIV/AIDS patients are much severe and may begin abruptly.

- Watery stool, diarrhea with or without blood, and stomach cramps.
- Mild fever and feeling of illness, muscle ache, and fatigue.
- Nausea, vomiting, and lack of appetite.
- Discomfort in the abdomen, feeling of gas, and audible rumbling.

## Diagnosis:

Diagnosis of diarrhea is obvious but the cause needs to be determined.

Your healthcare provider may request one or more stool samples for laboratory analysis. Presence of white blood cells and oocytes confirms cryptosporidiosis.

## Treatment:

There are no specific drugs or medications used to remedy cryptosporidiosis. Usually medications are prescribed to alleviate diarrhea and fever. Increased water/fluid intake is recommended for eventual cure.

## Prevention:

People with HIV must take preventive measures and additional precautions to be free of cryptosporidiosis. A few recommended tips to avoid infection are listed below.

- Drink only boiled, bottled, or filtered water.
- Consume only properly cooked food. If raw fruits, vegetables, and salads are on your menu thoroughly wash them before enjoying a bite.
- Thoroughly wash hands before and after visiting rest room.
- Wash hands and any part of your body that may come into contact with diapers, soiled linen, and stool.
- Avoid intimate sexual contact/practices that may result in hand or mouth exposure to fecal matter.
- Exposure to cattle, farm animals, stray cats, and dogs must be limited. If you must be around animals and cannot avoid proximity or exposure take precautions - wear gloves and mask. When done promptly change clothes, thoroughly wash hands with soap and water, or better still take a shower.

## HIV/AIDS and Cancer

Several types of cancers are common among HIV/AIDS patients because of compromised immune response. A weak immune system can afford only a weak response and inadequate protection to HIV/AIDS victims. HIV and cancer causing viruses further weaken immune barriers, provide greater opportunity to grow and spread cancers in the body. Such viruses also promote opportunistic infections in HIV/AIDS patients. Some such common viruses are listed below.

- Epstein - Barr virus (EBV)
- Hepatitis B virus
- Hepatitis C virus
- Herpes simplex virus (1&2)
- Human papillomavirus (HPV)

HIV positive habitual smokers are at higher risk for several types of cancers. Risk for lung disease such as TB, histoplasmosis, pneumonia, MAC, and toxoplasmosis is also high.

Greater awareness, prompt diagnosis, and improved care have contributed to quality life and longevity for many HIV/AIDS patients. This has also increased risk for acquiring OIs and variety of cancers. This situation is unavoidable as all HIV/AIDS people, though "healthy" still deal with compromised immune system.

Some of the common cancers and conditions for HIV/AIDS are listed below.

- Invasive cervical cancer: Cervical cancer caused by HPV.
- Kaposi sarcoma: Herpes virus causes Kaposi sarcoma. Kaposi sarcoma of the throat and lungs can be fatal.
- Non - Hodgkin lymphoma is caused by Epstein - Bar virus. The virus usually infects lymph nodes in the neck, arm pits, groin, and inside the stomach.
- HIV/AIDS is also known to cause bone and joint problems, neurological disorders, nutritional inconvenience, pain, and wasting syndrome.

## Prognosis:

Advances in medical research and technology have brought hope and promise to victims of AIDS. The status marked for death is changed sure to live. Decreased death rate among HIV/AIDS patients is the direct result of greater awareness, education, advanced technology, and improved all-round healthcare. This trend will continue as communities work together, devise ways to cope with the current situation, and eventually beat the odds. More needs to be done to create awareness, value, and rewards of prevention. Avoiding risk factors and seeking prompt medical care must be a priority. However hereditary and genetic factors are beyond our control.

## Life with HIV/AIDS

Modern medicine and current advances in treatment with new and potent drugs has helped thousands of HIV patients. People seeking medical advice are living longer and healthier. Availability of multiple support systems, better care, and education has contributed heavily to promote quality life and healthy living.

Most people infected by HIV eventually develop AIDS if not treated and managed. Time interval between infection and eventual AIDS is dependent upon several factors such as:

- Hereditary (genetics)
- Age
- Nutrition
- Good hygiene
- Overall living conditions and quality medical care.

Stress, depression, anxiety, and lack of medical care may shorten the time interval between HIV and AIDS.

## Tips to Live "Healthy" with HIV:

- Persons living with HIV need much compassion, emotional support, and above all skilled medical care.
- Primary and specialized healthcare providers and considerate family and friends can make a difference.
- Specialists in the U.S. have the experience, aware of current treatment techniques, willing to listen, understand, guide, and articulate.
- Prompt and meticulous adherence to treatment plan can produce favorable outcome.
- If medications adversely affect, make you ill, call your doctor, follow suggestions, and keep notes.
- Healthy sexual behavior, safe sex practices, and disease free partner selection help reduce risk of reinfection.
- Drugs, alcohol, and smoking can aggravate HIV and other co-infections. Consider kicking the habit for your good health.
- Immunization (s) for opportunistic infections, hepatitis (A&B), and other STDs such as HPV should be considered.
- Regular exercise, healthy diet, and overall better care may enhance immune system and reduce risk for opportunistic infections.

There may be many more ways to protect from risk factors. Patients must consult specialists and follow advice. Personal and professional interests must be considered in devising a holistic approach for better living. Following activities and suggestions may be helpful:

- Join groups and organizations that promote overall awareness and healthy living with HIV/AIDS.
- Seek and offer support to fellow patients. Open communication eases anxiety, improves understanding, and above all it can be a morale booster.
- Candid discussion of health-related issues may help ease anxiety, depression, and pain.
- Sharing experience, tips to improve quality healthy living may add even more fun.
- Look for public or group events and activities to learn more.
- Local library, newspapers, radio, Red Cross, and TV are a good resource.

## Coping With AIDS

People diagnosed with HIV must deal with scores of issues affecting their health, family, social/professional obligations, and fight life-threatening illness at the same time – a huge challenge. Emotional, mental, psychological, and personal problems result in anger, depression, helplessness, stress, and frustration. Insecurity and bleak future in the horizon is a true reality for many. Most HIV patients feel stigmatized therefore stay away from public eye. No book or guide of this kind can adequately address all such issues, therefore patients and their well -wishers must seek helpful information from their trusted family physician. Family physician may recommend:

- Major adaptive changes based on personal/ professional situation.
- Practical ways to cope with illness by suggesting strategies best for your life-style.
- Behavioral changes to protect self, family, and sex partners from HIV and other common STDs.
- Assistance with reproductive choices, gaining access to health care, changes in personal relationships, and overcome social stigmatization.
- Behavioral and psychological services to beat depression.
- Importance of medical compliance, follow-up care, partner notification, and risk reduction.

Besides your family physician other valuable sources listed below can also help.

Friends and church groups

Personal counselor/group therapists

Hospital based out-reach services

Local Red Cross

Social services/community services

Local public/private library

Any/all organizations that support, counsel, and care for HIV/AIDS patients

## 2. Genital Warts - Condyloma acuminata and Cervical Cancer Human Papillomavirus – HPV

Human Papillomavirus, a sexually transmitted DNA tumor virus can cause warts in or around vagina, rectum, and penis among sexually active women and men. In the U.S., more than 50% of sexually active men and women acquire at least one anogenital HPV infection with warts. As such more than 6.5 million Americans become infected each year. More than 20 million Americans aged 15 – 50 years are currently HPV positive and the number is steadily growing.

HPV infection may also indicate immune compromised status of the patient. Recurring and persistent oncogenic HPV infection(s) though transient may signal strong risk for development of pre-cancers and cancers among men and women.

More than 100 different HPV types are currently known. Most HPV types are harmless but about 40 virus types cause epithelial and cutaneous abnormalities such as genital warts and cancers. Most sexually active men and women from all walks of life, age, education, socioeconomic background, and sexual orientation can acquire HPV. Some low risk HPV (non-oncogenic) types can cause tiny bumps, flat raised warts, and wart clusters anywhere on the body. Genital warts are a cause of bother, cosmetically unsightly, and can get co-infected by bacteria or yeast if picked or scratched. High risk HPV (HR-HPV) types 16, 18, 31 and 45 are associated with 70 - 80% cancers of the cervix and intraepithelial neoplasms of the anus, rectum, penis, urethra, vagina, mouth, throat, and esophagus.

## Risk for HPV – Who is at greater risk?

Most men rarely experience serious health concerns due to HPV but few may develop genital warts and cancer of the penis. Penile cancer is rare among circumcised men but is a concern for uncircumcised men. However for young sexually active women cervical cancer can be fatal. Studies indicate risk is much greater for young than older women aged over 40 years.

- Young (less than 25 years) woman are at higher risk for HPV types 16, 18, 31 and 45 to genital warts and cervical cancer.
- Studies have shown that young girls (less than16 years) exposed to early (first) sexual experience with intercourse are at greater risk.
- Sexual intercourse with persons who have/had multiple sex partners and commercial sex workers increase risk.
- Most college students who entertain multiple sex partners are at higher risk.
- Sexual promiscuity/behavior is also a high risk factor for most men and women.
- Anogenital warts with high and low risk HPV are common among MSM and WSW. Anal cancer among MSM is common.
- Immune compromised persons such as HIV positive men and women have a much higher rate of HPV incidence. This population is also known to have much larger warts with longer episodes of the disease that is less responsive to treatment.

## Transmission of HPV:

HPV is transmitted by intimate person to person skin contact - usually during sexual intercourse. Some infected persons may not have visible warts on the genitals therefore sex-partners have no way of knowing the disease status of their new-found love or old flame. Virus usually gains entry to the host through mucous membrane of the vagina or cervix among women. For men, the virus finds its way through penis, scrotum, anus, and rectum.

An infected person can transmit HPV as described below:

- Genital - genital contact with or without penetration, manual – genital, oral – genital, and oral - anal.
- Genital HPV is very common among (more than 50%) homosexual men and women.
- HPV can be transmitted by sex toys, clothing, and other objects but actual viral transmission via this route is questionable.
- HPV is not transmitted to the baby through breast milk.

## Transmission Prevention:

Transmission and infection of HPV and other sexually transmitted infections (STIs) can be prevented with greater awareness and education among girls, women, and men who are at higher risk of acquiring STIs. A few proven ways to prevent HPV are listed below.

- Best way to prevent HPV and STIs is to abstain from sex or have sex with an uninfected person who practices monogamy.
- Avoid sexual relationship with persons with anogenital warts and lesions.
- Currently two FDA approved vaccines are available, quadrivalent Gardasil and bivalent Cervarix. Vaccines can protect against most common HPV infections that cause anogenital warts and cervical cancer.
- Administered as directed Gardasil can protect recipients against four HPV strains 6, 11, 16, and 18 and Cervarix against 16 and 18.
- For vaccine to be effective all three doses should be received before (preferably) exposure to the virus types causing HPV warts and cancer.
- Regular screening (pap-smear test) and follow-up procedures (if indicated) can prevent some cervical cancers.
- Early detection may help resolve symptoms and prevent cervical cancer in most women.
- Condom use may lower risk for some but not all. Condom must be used all the time – the right way. Condom does not protect groin, lower abdomen, and thighs.
- Genital washing, douching, and urination after sex will not lower risk.

## Symptoms:

HPV infection in most sexually active men and women can be asymptomatic. Therefore newly acquired infection can go completely unnoticed. And then, if visible bumps or warts, itching, pain, or fever do appear months after exposure such symptoms may be difficult to associate with HPV. For some warts may appear immediately after exposure only to disappear within weeks. This false "feeling free and safe" of infection by HPV creates a false sense of security as a result most people are likely to ignore HPV exposure altogether. Asymptomatic infection by high risk HPV in some women can cause genital warts and changes to the genital epithelial surface weeks after exposure eventually resulting in cervical cancer.

However in an ideal HPV infection tiny bumps may appear anytime between 1- 6 months post exposure. Genital warts usually develop on warm, moist areas such as genitals. Some common symptoms are listed below.

- In most women usually tiny, dark, or dark brown warts appear around the anus, vagina, vaginal skin, or vulva. Warts may also develop on the cervix and inner labia.
- In men warts appear slightly below the foreskin (if uncircumcised) or on the penile head or shaft. Warts may also appear on the scrotum.
- Uncircumcised men may notice tiny flat warts inside the foreskin causing itching, discomfort, and redness of foreskin.

- Some men may notice tiny flat warts inside the urethral opening. This may cause sharp pain, bleeding, and urethral discharge.
- In men and women warts may appear just below the genitals and anus or both. This is most common among homosexual men and women who engage in anal sex.
- The size, shape, and number of warts may wary among individuals. Sometimes tiny warts may grow into small or large clusters resembling cauliflower.
- Slightly raised fleshy warts are harder than the surrounding skin, may or may not itch, but bleed if picked.
- Warts are usually painless and may go unnoticed. Careful periodic visual examination and touch/feeling of genitals (in private) is recommended.
- Immune impaired persons usually experience severe symptoms with larger warts.

In most people warts disappear without treatment but most HIV positive persons require prolonged treatment.

Like any other viral infection HPV no matter the type can be transient. But for some people for unknown reasons infection tend to linger on. The virus may be contained but not conquered. Infected persons may have had their warts excised, burnt, or treated but the virus persists in the host for life. At an opportune time the virus may re-infect with distinct visible symptoms - this is known as reactivation. People once infected by family of HPV types rarely experience re-infection.

## Diagnosis:

- Genital warts are diagnosed by visual inspection of the infected area (s) such as mouth, throat, vulva, vagina, cervix, penis, and anus.
- A careful pelvic and rectal examination is performed. A cervical scrapping or swab may be taken (even if the person is asymptomatic) for Hybrid Capture 2 HPV DNA test. The genetic material of the virus is identified to confirm the presence of low risk types or high risk types (16 and 18) of HPV.
- Tiny, flat bumps on cervix confirm infection in most cases. When such bumps cannot be seen with the naked eye and HPV DNA test is positive, a procedure called colposcopy is performed to examine the cervix. Procedure provides a magnified view of the cervical wall hence even tiny warts can be detected.
- Colposcopy enables the detection of mild, moderate, or severe dysplasia or degree (grades 2 or 3) of cervical intraepithelial neoplasia (CIN).
- Most men and women regardless of their sexual orientation are routinely examined for genital warts. HPV types 6 and 11 selectively target anus and genitals.
- Healthcare providers also carefully examine around and inside the mouth for HPV warts.
- HPV DNA test is not recommended for males simply because of lack of utility. HPV is common in men. Some may have genital warts but

HPV triggered penile cancer is extremely rare in circumcised men.

- Biopsy can confirm genital warts but visual inspection is adequate. Physicians rarely recommend routine biopsy other than for extraordinary medical reasons.
- Pap-smear test can identify women at risk or imminent risk based on epithelial cellular changes.

For most viral infections, reliable screening and confirmatory diagnostic tests are performed however for a specific type of HPV infection a reliable serologic blood test is not available.

## Testing for Genital HPV Infection:

HPV DNA test, only FDA approved procedure for high risk HPV is currently used to detect cervical cancer. Cervical scrapping of infected, suspected, and well women is secured for testing. DNA test is a valuable screening tool that can also determine whether or not high risk patient(s) has developed cancerous or pre-cancerous lesions of the cervix since the last pelvic examination.

HPV DNA testing has no diagnostic value for men and should not be used to determine current status of genital warts or HPV infection. HPV is not routinely cultured or serologically tested in the laboratory for identification and confirmation of infection.

## Treatment:

No known treatment is currently available to eradicate HPV. Only symptoms and disorders caused by HPV such as genital warts and cancers can be treated. HPV remains in the body even after treatment.

Genital warts can be irritating, annoying, and to most infected persons cosmetically unacceptable. If not treated, warts may resolve within weeks or remain the same in size and number for a long time. Invasive treatment and therapy may get rid of the symbolic nuisance temporarily (only to reappear weeks or months later) but not the infection itself. Therefore when confronted with such a trivial situation see your healthcare provider, look for a second opinion (if you must) in order to arrive at an informed medical decision. Genital warts may disappear (in some people) with no treatment - you may want to wait out.

The treatment options described below are mainly cosmetic. Ugly warts can be surgically excised only to reappear.

## Topical Treatment:

Your healthcare provider may prescribe cream, gel, ointment, or solution for treatment. Dosage and frequency for application may vary. Location, age, and size of warts may determine best treatment management option(s).

**Podophyllin** (Podofilox (0.5% solution or gel) is recommended for external warts only. Solution or gel is applied to the warts directly. Podophyllin is also available in cream form.

**Trichloracetic acid** (TCA) solution is available to treat internal (inner labia, urethra, and vagina) and external warts. Solution applied as directed, may clear the visible warts but tend to recur in some people.

**Imiquimod** cream (5%) is prescribed to treat external genital warts. Creams are much easier to apply than solutions.

Sinecatechins 15% ointment is yet another available treatment option. Size and location of wart(s) determines frequency of application.

## Some provider administered procedures are listed below:

1. **Cryotherapy**: External warts are subjected to freezing temperatures for a short time. The procedure destroys warts.
2. **Surgery**: Area around warts to be excised is numbed and warts excised with a scalpel.
3. **Electro- surgery**: Local anesthetic is applied around the warts. Warts are then excised with an electric blade.
4. **Laser surgery**: A laser beam is directed on the wart (s). This procedure is expensive and requires specialized skill.

Most people experience frequent recurrence of genital warts requiring repeated treatment. Though most people may respond well to above treatment (s) some may not, therefore patients must monitor their progress or lack there off closely. Always rely on your doctor's advice for favorable results. Uncircumcised men can prevent painful wart recurrence inside the foreskin by opting for circumcision.

## Follow - Up:
Annual screening or repeat procedure is not recommended for women aged >30 years of age with normal HR-HPV (high risk HPV) and Pap tests. This interval can be increased to 3 years.

However women with abnormal results require additional follow – up procedures such as colposcopic examination, biopsy if indicated, and repeat pap-smears in 12 and 24 months. Such high risk patients are referred to specialists for state of the art aggressive management and care.

For women aged >21years with abnormal HR-HPV and pap-smear results, following options are recommended:

- Colposcopy
- Repeat pap-smear at 6 and 12 months
- HR-HPV DNA screening

Above procedures provide useful information and determine additional treatment options. Specialists must be consulted in order to provide needful skilled care.

Among women aged <21 years high risk HPV infections usually heal rapidly but repeat pap-tests should be recommended at 12 and 24 months to monitor progress.

However abnormal Pap test results must be followed up by colposcopy and other procedures as described already.

## Management of Sex Partners:

Patients' past and present sex partners should be identified, examined, diagnosed, counseled, and treated for HPV if indicated. Benefits of risk reduction techniques and proper condom use should also be discussed. Condom use by male sex partners of sexually active women can reduce risk for cervical cancer, HPV infection, and can help heal existing infection faster.

Index patient and sex partners should be (if appropriate) informed about newly approved HPV quadrivalent

Gardasil and bivalent Cervarix vaccines. Men and women who meet required criteria are offered age appropriate regimen as per guidelines. Both FDA approved vaccines have great promise, hope, and value for millions of men and women worldwide.

## HPV and Cervical Cancer

HR-HPV infection is likely to result in cervical cancer if not diagnosed and treated early. Prevention of this deadly disease is possible. Therefore early detection, treatment, and management are critically important. Many women still die from cervical cancer each year in the U.S.; such fatalities can be prevented if routinely screened and managed as recommended by experts.

HPV (types 16 and 18) infection increases risk for anal and cervical cancers among men and women. Even though this number is small, it is wise to avoid such risk altogether. Safe sex along with risk free behavior can prevent STIs. Risk (s) for cancer and serious complications can be avoided by immunization as directed by healthcare givers.

Most healthcare providers in the U.S. recommend annual pelvic examination and pap- smear test for women. Pap test detects changes in the composition and complexion of cervical cells. Physicians can promptly evaluate such patients and initiate appropriate treatment and follow up care.

Immunization as indicated can prevent HPV infection, warts, and cancers among men and women. Currently two such vaccines, Gardasil and Cervarix are approved by FDA to provide life-saving benefits.

## Prevention of Cervical Cancer

Only 50 years ago more women died from cervical cancer than any other type of cancer in the United States. Worldwide figures may be mindboggling. In the U.S., annual death rate has decreased markedly in the last 40 years due to widespread cervical cancer screening (pap-test) and aggressive treatment of pre-cancerous conditions caused by HPV.

FDA approved quadrivalent HPV vaccine (June, 2006) also known as Gardasil for virus types 6, 11, 16, and 18 developed by Merck & company offers great promise and hope for thousands of sexually active and to be active men and women. Cervarix, another FDA approved (Oct. 2009) bivalent vaccine for HPV types (16 and 18) developed by Glaxo Smith Kline Laboratories is also available. Vaccine is prepared from non-infectious viral particles and administered in three doses intramuscularly over a six month period at 0, 2, and 6 month intervals.

Vaccine administered to young girls (teen and pre-teen) and women (ages 13- 26) can protect against the four types of HPV that cause 70% of cervical cancers. Gardasil is also recommended for boys and men (ages 9-26) that cause 90% of genital warts. Bivalent vaccine will protect against HR-HPV types 16 and 18. Availability, demography, and age may dictate Gardasil or Cervarix prescription.

## Vaccination Recommendations:

- Vaccine is recommended for girls 9 – 12 years of age.
- 13 – 26 year old girls/women can be vaccinated if not received all the three doses.

- Those who received 1st dose only should be given 2nd and 3rd doses for compliance.
- For best results girls/women should receive the full vaccine regimens before engaging in serious sexual activity.
- Vaccine is most effective to virus types they are not yet exposed.
- Vaccine is 100% effective in preventing genital warts and cancers of the cervix, vagina, and vulva in girls and women who have not been infected.
- Vaccine can prevent 90% of genital warts among boys and men administered as indicated.
- Vaccine may cause mild redness/soreness at the site of injection. Other adverse effects include (a) fainting spells in rare cases and (b) skin disorders such as itching and burning for some but no fatalities have been reported yet.

Quadrivalent or bivalent vaccine is also recommended for boys and men ages 9-26 years. Vaccine is effective to the HPV virus types that they are not yet exposed. Vaccinated boys and men fail to acquire cancer inducing HPV types therefore cannot transmit infection nor induce cancers to their sex partners.

All vaccinated girls and women must take their genital health seriously. All sexually active girls and women require regular/periodic pap-tests (annual or once in three years) as cancer/genital warts screening tool. Abnormal cell changes can be detected early and treated before progressing into cancer.

Much research, discussion, and debate has confirmed safety and efficacy of vaccines for boys, men, girls, and women. HPV vaccines don't cure genital warts and cervical cancer – but immunize, protect, and prevent acquisition of the disease for life.

## 3. Hepatitis A, B, and C Viral Infections Vaccine Preventable STDs

Hepatitis causes inflammation of the liver - one of body's major organs located in the upper abdomen. Common cause of hepatitis is a group of viruses, specifically viruses A, B, C, D, E, F, and G. These are known to target the liver causing infection and inflammation that is named after each virus. Liver infections are also caused by cytomegalovirus (CMV), Epstein-Barr virus (EBV), and arbovirus (yellow fever). Other main causes of liver disease are alcohol and drugs.

Hepatitis can be acute or chronic. Acute viral hepatitis may last for less than 6 months but chronic hepatitis may linger on for life.

Hepatitis is a global problem. Unsafe water supplies, inadequate sewer system, below standard health care have contributed heavily to exasperate already existing problem into a crisis.

The scope of this guide is limited to STDs frequently caused by hepatitis viruses A, B, and C. Hepatitis A and B viral infections can be prevented by vaccination. Research is underway to develop an effective vaccine for hepatitis C.

# Hepatitis A
## Hepatitis A Virus – HAV

Hepatitis A is a common food/waterborne liver infection caused by Hepatitis A (HAV) virus. Hepatitis A outbreak is a result of poor personal hygiene, untreated drinking water, lack of sanitation and sewer systems. Frequent hepatitis A outbreaks are perennial problems in many poor and developing countries. Most such countries frequently experience hepatitis A outbreaks as a direct result of inadequate clean drinking water, contaminated food supply, and unsafe sewer system. Hepatitis A incidence in the United States is not common but increased international travel, house-hold contacts, playmates, accidents, and floods have increased the risk. U.S. health agencies reported 996 active cases of hepatitis A in 2010.

HAV infects and replicates in the liver causing a self-limited acute syndrome that does not progress into chronic liver disease. HAV incubates in the liver for approximately 30 -40 days post-exposure then shed in large quantities with feces. Hepatitis A can relapse in some people, especially persons >40 years of age within six months after the initial incident.

## Transmission of HAV:
HAV can be transmitted as follows:

- Fecal-oral route during intimate sexual activity. Oral-anal contact and oral-genital contact are two primary means of HAV transmission.

- Sexual transmission of the virus can be a behavioral issue for many. Persons engaged in oral - anal intercourse, rimming, anal stimulation are at high risk.
- Sharing food, drinks, water, and utensils with infected persons is a leading cause of non-sexual transmission of HAV.
- Raw shellfish and oyster lovers are at higher risk for hepatitis A infection.
- HAV is occasionally detected in saliva of infected persons but transmission of virus by saliva is very rare.
- Infected persons' blood and saliva are not known to transmit hepatitis A.
- HAV is extremely hardy and can survive outside the host for several months. This increases risk for transmission.

## Prevention of HAV Transmission:

Efforts must be made to prevent HAV transmission by eliminating risk factors. A few practical tips to avoid conventional and accidental hepatitis A infection are listed below:

- Vaccination for hepatitis A will prevent infection. Vaccine is given in two doses (IM) at 0 and 6-12 months. Vaccine is good for life.
- Most healthcare providers in the U.S. recommend new combined hepatitis A and B vaccine to prospective candidates.
- If you believe that you are exposed to hepatitis A for whatever reason talk to your healthcare provider ASAP. Intramuscular (IM) immu-

noglobulin (IG) administered within 2 weeks post exposure can prevent nearly 85% of new HAV episodes.

- Elderly persons and people over age 40 usually do not require vaccine. More than 75% elderly men and women are immune for hepatitis A. However in emergency situations immunoglobulin can be administered.
- Sexual transmission of HAV can be prevented by avoiding oral- anal contact.
- Condom use may prevent other STDs but not hepatitis A.
- Good personal hygiene is important to prevent transmission of hepatitis A.
- Sharing utensils, cups, glasses, and food with persons of unknown health status must be avoided as a precaution
- Thoroughly wash hands with soap and warm water before and after visits to the restroom.
- Kitchen personnel must be extra careful when handling raw food, fruits, and vegetables. Follow guidelines set forth by the local health department.
- Restaurant employees must wash hands and change uniform often especially after rest room visits.
- Consume only heated, temperature controlled, and safety inspected food especially meat and fish products.
- Raw fruit and veggies are healthy but wash them thoroughly before consumption.

- Food counter, cutting board, utensils, and cooking accessories must be washed with disinfectants, soap, warm, and hot water before and after use.
- People working with children (daycare) must take extra precautions. Diapers, soiled linen, and towels must be handled as per OSHA guidelines.
- Nursing and affiliated staff in adult care, hospitals, nursing homes, and senior citizen centers must frequently wash hands, especially between patients.
- Patient's stool, urine, sputum, blood, and clothing must be handled with extreme care – as per universal precautions and OSHA guidelines.
- Public toilets and other common places are also a matter of concern. Infected persons may have not cleaned or improperly used the facilities.

Persons at high risk such as (listed below) should be offered pre-exposure hepatitis A vaccine or post exposure immunoglobulin. All healthcare professionals, auxiliary medical staff, and employees for institutionalized living must consider immunization for HAV and HBV.

A. Homosexual men (MSM) and lesbian women.
B. Habitual drug users (injection and non-injection drug use).
C. Persons with known chronic liver disease (CLD).
D. Persons with hepatitis B and C.
E. Victims of sexual assault and physical abuse.
F. All health care givers and auxiliary medical staff listed above.

## Symptoms for Hepatitis A:

Most adults and children rarely develop symptoms for hepatitis A. Most adults who develop any symptoms do so suddenly between 2 - 6 weeks after exposure. Some common symptoms are listed below.

- Poor appetite, nausea, and vomiting.
- Dehydration.
- Feeling feverish, malaise, and fatigue.
- Muscle and joint ache, headache, and pain in the upper abdomen due to liver inflammation.
- Mild to severe diarrhea, jaundice, darkening of urine, and pale stool.
- Some may experience sore throat and itchy skin.
- Most symptoms disappear within 6-8 weeks. These symptoms rarely reappear. Acute hepatitis A is rarely fatal and most likely never chronic.

## Diagnosis:

Acute viral hepatitis A is suspected based on symptoms just described. Physical examination may reveal jaundice and tender/enlarged liver. Special blood tests are necessary to determine current status of infection.

- Elevated liver enzymes suggest acute hepatitis A
- Presence of IgM in blood suggest current acute infection
- Presence of total anti – HAV antibodies indicates past exposure or immunity

- Antibody (IG) blood test is performed to distinguish liver infections such as Hepatitis A, B, C, mononucleosis, and influenza.
- Alcohol and drug induced hepatitis is confirmed if blood is negative for viral antibodies.

## Treatment:

Seriously ill and dehydrated persons may require hospitalization for intravenous (IV) therapy, and plenty of bed rest. Patients with severe nausea and vomiting may be at risk for liver failure. In most cases fluids, anti-nausea medications, and bed rest are recommended for speedy recovery. Appetite will soon return jaundice will fade away within 8 -10 weeks, and liver function tests eventually become normal.

## Post Exposure Prophylactic Treatment:

People suspecting recent exposure to HAV can avoid risk for acute hepatitis by visiting their healthcare provider or clinic ASAP. Nature and circumstances of an exposure dictate necessary treatment. If previously vaccinated for HAV an additional dose of IG or vaccine may be administered.

- Usually HAV specific (single-antigen) vaccine or immunoglobulin (IG) is administered intramuscularly.
- For healthy persons (< 40 years of age) single-antigen vaccine (age appropriate) is recommended over IG. Vaccine has life - long benefits.
- People > 40 years of age and those with impaired immune system such as HIV/AIDS and chronic liver disease (CLD) require care-

ful evaluation – vaccine or IG may be selected based on patient history and current health status.

- For persons > 40 years of age usually IG is the shot of choice over vaccine.
- Immune compromised persons may not respond well to HAV vaccine due to poor immune response.
- In some unique situations such as sexual assault, abuse, and accidental exposure persons may be administered HAV vaccine and IG simultaneously. However vaccine recipients must get the remainder booster shots for lasting benefits.

## Pre-Exposure Vaccination:

Pre-exposure vaccine is recommended to people who seek incidental and accidental protection from HAV. Health conscious people must follow their personal physician's advice. Pre-exposure vaccination can prevent Hep A among following groups of people who are at much higher risk:

- All health care personnel.
- People employed in daycare, detention centers, group homes, hospitals, and institutions such as correctional facilities, prisons etc.
- Newly diagnosed HIV patient(s).
- Drug users sharing needles.
- Homosexual men and women.
- Persons diagnosed with CLD.
- Persons with chronic HBV and HCV.

## Prognosis:

People with acute hepatitis A usually resolve infection within 4 - 8 weeks, many on their own and some with supportive therapy described above. Hepatitis A is very rarely fatal and does not progress into chronic syndrome. People previously infected or vaccinated for hepatitis A will be positive for specific antibodies for life therefore are protected against hepatitis A for life.

## Hepatitis B
## Hepatitis B Virus – HBV

Hepatitis B is a very common blood-borne disease that causes inflammation of the liver resulting in chronic self-limited hepatitis, cirrhosis, and even cancer in some patients. Chronic hepatitis is much milder than the acute form of the disease but can persist for years. If not treated chronic hepatitis B can progress into cirrhosis or hepatocellular cancer (HCC). HBV is present in high concentration in blood and to lesser extent in body fluids of infected people. Body fluids such as semen, vaginal secretions, saliva, blood, and wound exudates can transmit hepatitis B to susceptible sex and needle sharing partners. In 2010, CDC reported 2042 new HBV infections in the U.S. HBV is a very serious health concern worldwide.

## Transmission:

Hepatitis B virus (HBV) is usually transmitted by infected persons to their sex and needle sharing partners. Many chronically ill people are carriers of hepatitis B virus but asymptomatic. HBV can be transmitted by carriers as described below.

- Infected persons can transmit HBV by unprotected sex.
- Exchange of body fluids such as blood, saliva, semen, and vaginal secretions can cause infection.
- People who have unprotected sex with multiple sex-partners present great risk of HBV transmission.
- Persons sharing needles for drug use are at greater risk. Body piercing and tattooing also can expose people to substantial risk.
- Blood donors with chronic hepatitis B infection (carriers) were major transmitters of HBV until a few decades ago. Screening of all blood and blood products have greatly reduced such risk.
- Accidental exposure to blood and body fluids from needle sticks, open wounds, and tear/break in the skin can cause hepatitis B.
- Accidental cut with soiled surgical tools can also cause infection.
- Pregnant women can infect fetus. This can happen in the womb or during normal child birth. Most such babies become carriers of HBV.
- Sexual assault and physical abuse can transmit HBV. Predators must be tested ASAP so victims receive prompt appropriate treatment.

## Prevention of HBV Transmission:

Prevention of HBV transmission can be accomplished with an effective strategy, coordination of resources, and communication. The plan must include healthcare providers, clinics, hospitals, and public officials. Following suggestions may help health conscious good Samaritans.

## 1. Hepatitis B immune globulin (HBIG) administered IM post exposure:

- HBIG is prepared from human plasma containing very high concentrations of HBV (surface antigen). HBIG provides temporary protection up to 6 months.
- HBIG is recommended for post exposure prophylactic (PEP) treatment as an adjunct to HBV vaccine or alone. Victims of sexual assault, abuse, accidents, and other forms of exposure can benefit from this treatment.

## 2. Hepatitis B vaccine:

- Hep B vaccine is used extensively to prevent HBV infection. In some situations immunoglobulin and vaccine are administered simultaneously for favorable outcome. Vaccine is normally administered at 0, 1, and 6 months. Vaccine can provide life-long protection.
- Vaccine is recommended for immunization and prophylaxis. Adolescents, adults, healthcare professionals, and general public must

be encouraged to be immunized for life-long protection.

- Persons entering group homes, retirement facilities, nursing homes, correctional institutions and prisons should be educated, screened for HBV, and immunized if indicated.
- Immunization is recommended for all pregnant women. Procedure will protect infants against hepatitis B.
- HIV positive persons may not respond well to Hep B vaccine, yet a modified dose is recommended to elicit better response.
- House hold contacts, needle sharing, and sex partners of persons with current HBV infection need to be identified and treated as indicated. Initial regimen and subsequent age appropriate vaccine or HBIG (or both) administered as per guidelines.

## 3. Precautions and counseling:

- HBV infected persons and their sex partners should be instructed to practice safe sex at all times to avoid consequences of risky reckless behavior.
- Needle sharing must be discouraged. Many cities and communities in the U.S. distribute free condoms and needles to habitual drug users.
- HBV positive persons must be advised to refrain from donating blood, blood products, semen, organs, and tissue.

- HBV infected persons must also avoid or limit alcohol intake. Alcohol affects liver function.
- Medications and drugs affecting liver must be discontinued for safer substitutes. Most health-care providers and pharmacists can guide patients.
- HBV infected persons must be advised to inform/remind their Hep B status to dentist and caregivers as a precaution.
- Hep B positive persons must not share personal items such as toothbrush, razor, nail cutter, and the like with anyone.
- Persons free of HBV should avoid sexual intercourse/intimacy with known needle sharing drug users and alcoholics (if possible).
- Support from family, friends, and community in general can help Hep B positive persons to cope with chronic infection.
- Washing genitals, hot/cold showers after sex does not prevent HBV.

## Symptoms:

Most people exposed to HBV become chronic with no symptoms. People who develop the characteristic symptoms may do so gradually within 6 weeks to 6 months therefore such mild symptoms may go completely unnoticed. In some people however symptoms listed below may appear within 6 – 12 weeks post exposure.

- Mild low grade fever, feeling of illness, fatigue, and joint pain.
- Poor appetite and nausea (rarely).

- Some people may develop itchy rashes on the skin.
- Pain in the upper abdomen due to enlarged (swollen) liver.
- Jaundice, coloring of urine (dark brown), and stool (pale white) develop eventually in severe cases.
- If not promptly managed acute hepatitis B may cause cirrhosis, chronic liver disease (CLD), hepatocellular carcinoma (HCC), liver failure, and death.
- People who survive acute hepatitis B may develop serious complications such as cirrhosis and hepatic carcinoma (liver cancer).
- People with chronic hepatitis B may also develop enlarged spleen, spider like veins, and fluid retention (kidney dis-function).
- Women with autoimmune hepatitis B are at risk for conditions such as acne, anemia, lung scarring, inflammation of kidneys and thyroid glands. In some women autoimmune condition may affect menstrual cycle.

Most symptoms described above may occur gradually and in some rare cases abruptly. When any such symptoms appear call your doctor ASAP to get tested for hepatitis A, B, and C.

## Diagnosis:

In the absence or presence of characteristic hepatitis B symptoms blood tests for liver function, HBV antigen and antibody are requested to determine patients' current health status. Recent infection can be confirmed by HBV antigen in blood. HBV antibody titer confirms past exposure and immunity to HBV.

- Presence of IgM to B core antigen (IgM anti-HBc) confirms recent acute HBV infection.
- Presence of antibody to HBsAg (anti HBs) indicates resolution and immunity for HBV.
- Presence of HBsAg and total anti-HBc, with IgM anti-HBc negative test confirms chronic hepatitis infection.

A biopsy may also be performed to determine mild or severe liver damage. Blood tests and biopsy results can determine an ideal effective strategy for care and treatment.

Liver function tests are routinely performed to evaluate and manage patients' response to treatment success.

HBV carriers should be tested for hepatitis D also known as delta hepatitis. Hepatitis B carriers are prone to delta hepatitis and can readily be super infected by hepatitis D. This dual attack may cause and hasten severe liver damage, cirrhosis, carcinoma, liver failure, and even death. Patients may also become active carriers of both hepatitis B and D. Such carriers are a huge risk to family, friends, and care givers.

## Treatment:

Healthcare providers and liver specialists usually provide only supportive treatment for patients with acute hepatitis B. But chronic form of the disease may require thorough evaluation and management by a liver specialist for CLD.

Besides professional therapeutic care for CLD patients are recommended bed rest, healthy diet, and most importantly abstinence from alcohol and drugs. Screening for hepato-cellular carcinoma (HCC) is also necessary.

Newly infected persons must seek medical advice promptly, preferably from a liver specialist. All options need to be carefully evaluated including best combination of medications, immunization, behavioral changes and alcohol/drug habit. Untreated hepatitis B can bring on severe consequences and eventual death.

## Pre-Exposure Vaccination:

Hepatitis B vaccination is recommended for all unvacci-nated adults and adolescents. Greater awareness of risk of infection may persuade most adults to seek protection from HBV. Special groups of people listed below should consider pre-exposure vaccination.

- All healthcare professionals, auxiliary, and sup-portive staff.
- Persons seeking treatment for HIV and com-mon STDs.
- Persons entering correctional facilities, deten-tion centers, and prisons.
- All employees of above facilities and support-ive personnel.
- Persons enlisted for drug abuse treatment.
- Adult care, Independent living, group homes, and Nursing home residents must seek medical advice concerning immunization.
- All adults/adolescents should seek vaccination as a preventive tool.

## Post-Exposure Prophylactic Treatment:

Accidental, unplanned, and unsolicited exposure to hepatitis B is an ongoing concern for all health care professionals. Hepatitis B is a serious occupational health hazard. Most victims of sexual assault and physical abuse are also at great risk for hepatitis B and other STDs. When encountered with a situation just described post-exposure prophylactic treatment is provided as described.

Hepatitis B vaccine and Hep B immunoglobulin (HBIG) can be administered for post-exposure prophylaxis. Vaccine is an active prophylactic agent whereas HBIG is considered passive. For certain emergency situations described below either both or only one (vaccine or HBIG) may be offered.

- Exposure to Hepatitis positive person (s) or a source (needle stick, surgical accident or infectious matter) is a serious health issue. Patient/victim must be promptly vaccinated and administered Immunoglobulin within 24 hours of exposure.
- Sexual contact or needle share with any hepatitis B positive person has great risk. Patient is promptly vaccinated and administered HBIG simultaneously at different sites.
- Victims of sexual assault and physical abuse by predators (s) who are positive for hepatitis B are treated with vaccine and Immunoglobulin at different sites.
- Victims of sexual assault and abuse by perpetrators of unknown hepatitis B status must be evaluated and vaccinated.

- Persons who accidentally come into contact with infectious matter, needle stick, bite, or exposures to blood/fluid of unknown HBV status are administered hepatitis B vaccine.

## Management of Hepatitis B Positive Persons:

Management of infected persons is a critical public health concern. Such people are at much higher risk to acquire common STDs and HIV. A well - conceived management strategy can ideally accomplish:

- Reduce/prevent new hepatitis B infections.
- Reduce/prevent other life-threatening infections.
- Protect infected persons from serious life-threatening co-infections and CLD.

These dual goals can be achieved with concerted effort by all concerned. A well co - ordinated partnership will pay heavy dividends. All state and local governments in the U.S. are well equipped to implement such a strategy. HBV positive persons need to be aware of the following:

- Healthcare providers, clinics, and testing facilities report hepatitis B antigen (HBsAg) positive persons to local or state health department.
- Hepatitis B positive persons should be routinely retested, chronic patients identified and referred to liver specialists for specialized care for CLD. Early intervention can save pain, suffering, and many lives.

- All members of the household, needle-sharing, and sex partners of chronic hepatitis B persons must be identified and treated as per guidelines. Sex and needle sharing partners must be instructed prevention methods and tools available such as vaccination, safe sex practices, free condom/needles (if available) and other barrier methods.
- Hepatitis B positive persons must be advised to take precautions and prevent transmission by practicing safe sex. Susceptible needle sharing and sex partners must be vaccinated.
- Hepatitis B positive persons must cover wounds, cuts, and skin lesions and lacerations at all times to prevent blood and fluid secretions.
- Refrain from donating blood, organs, tissue, plasma, platelets, and semen.
- Avoid sharing personal items such as nail cutters, razors, tooth-brush, needles, and any item contaminated by blood or body secretions.
- When seeking medical, dental, or any intrusive procedure (s) inform care givers your hepatitis B positive status.
- Hepatitis B infected persons must follow medical advice for good health for self, family, friends, needle sharing, and sex partners. Avoid alcohol consumption, drugs, and any substance that may adversely affect liver.
- Hepatitis B positive persons must also receive vaccination for hepatitis A to prevent or arrest liver disease.

Most HBV positive persons can enjoy normal living. Following useful information may help overcome prevailing apprehensions concerning hepatitis B positive people:

- Friends and family can help chronic hepatitis B persons cope with stress and anxiety by providing support and compassionate counseling – only when appropriate.
- Hepatitis B is NOT spread by coughing, hugging, physical contact, sharing food, beverages, utensils, and water fountains.

Hepatitis B patients can also get much needed help and support from local and community support groups. Information and activities of such groups may be available at clinics, doctor's office, hospitals, local library, Red-Cross, newspapers, radio, and television.

## Hepatitis C
## Hepatitis C Virus – HCV

Hepatitis C is a very common chronic blood-borne liver disease caused by HCV. Hepatitis C virus was known as non-A, non-B hepatitis before the discovery of the virus itself. Hepatitis C is prevalent worldwide. Approximately 3.2 million people are infected in the U. S. alone. Most HCV infected persons are at greater risk for chronic liver disease (CLD), HIV, and cancer of the liver.

There are several types of HCV viruses. The genetic differences among these viruses obviously influence degree and severity of infection but not the symptoms if any. Response to medications may vary among different types of HCV. Most common viral types in the U. S. are Type 1 (a, & b), 2, and 3. Occasionally other types such as 4, 5, 7, 8, and 9 are also identified in the U. S. This is mainly due to travel and interaction with people from other continents. 507 new hepatitis C infections were reported in the U.S. in 2010.

## Transmission:

HCV infected persons are a steady source of virus transmission to their sex partners, house hold contacts, friends, and family. Most infected people are asymptomatic therefore unaware of their illness hence unknowingly transmit HCV. Some methods of viral transmission are listed below.

- Recipients of un-scanned blood, blood products, hemodialysis, heart, kidney, and tissue transplants in the past (before 1992) were at high risk for hepatitis C infection.
- Drug users, especially those sharing needles are still at high risk. Tattooing with contaminated needles increases risk for HCV.
- Sexual transmission of hepatitis C is not very common yet it's still a problem to deal with. Intimate sexual contact, exchange of blood, saliva, semen, and vaginal secretions can potentially transmit hepatitis C.
- Pregnant women can infect the newborn before or during childbirth.

- Occupational health hazards for healthcare personnel may cause HCV transmission through body fluids.
- Accidental cuts with soiled equipment, needles, and objects can cause hepatitis C.
- Victims of sexual assault, abuse, and physical violence are at greater risk.

## Prevention of HCV Transmission:

At present no vaccine or immunoglobulin is available for HCV immunization or prophylaxis. Therefore healthcare professionals face the difficult task of reducing new transmissions, CLD, and other chronic infections. Current HCV management techniques include:

## 1. Identify HCV infected persons in the community.

- Provide counseling, medical treatment, and antiviral therapy, if indicated.
- Persons entertaining multiple sex partners, HIV positive men, and women are encouraged to practice safe sex.
- Drug users by needle sharing are at much higher risk for HIV and HCV.

Many HIV infected patients are also co-infected with HCV, a very deadly combination. Follow-up, professional counseling and testing may offer some hope and help reduce HCV transmission in this category of people.

## 2. Routine HCV testing and counseling be offered to persons such as:

- Blood and tissue recipients prior 1992.
- Recipients of clotting factor concentrate prior 1987.
- Long-term dialysis candidates.
- Persons with characteristic symptoms of liver disease.
- Children born to HCV positive women.
- All HIV positive and AIDS patients.

## 3. HCV infected persons should be advised:

- Not to donate blood, organs, tissue, skin, or semen.
- Not to share personal items such as toothbrush, razor, nail clippers etc.
- Avoid alcohol and drug use.
- Avoid medications/drugs that may further damage liver – talk to your doctor or pharmacist.

### Symptoms:

Most infected people are asymptomatic therefore most likely to ignore mild symptoms if any. Those who sense some discomfort may begin to feel symptoms 4-6 weeks after exposure. Symptoms for new infections may be much severe than those for reinfections. Some of the common symptoms are listed below.

- Mild fever, fatigue, and abdominal pain.
- Loss of appetite, feeling of nausea, and vomiting.

- Some may develop mild jaundice, discoloration of urine and stool.

Ignoring symptoms can lead to serious health problems involving liver. Infected people with or without symptoms respond differently - some resolve infection and develop immunity to HCV. But many develop chronic form of hepatitis C. Older people usually experience rapid progression of Hep C. Severe liver damage, jaundice, and complications can be fatal.

People with chronic hepatitis C regardless of their age need skilled professional care preferably from liver specialists. Excessive use of alcohol, medications, and substance abuse may accelerate serious life threatening episodes such as chronic liver disease (CLD), cirrhosis, liver cancer, liver failure, and even death.

## Diagnosis:

Hepatitis C active infection can be asymptomatic. Most infected persons may be unaware of nursing an infection much less suspect one. However people who engage in risky behaviors such as needle share, multiple sex partners, and all who suspect hepatitis C should visit their physicians or clinic for help. Patient history, sex and drug habits, along with symptoms if any will be documented. If hepatitis C is suspected diagnostic tests may be requested to confirm infection. HIV positive persons are routinely tested for HCV in the U.S.

1. **Antibody Test (EIA):** Presence of antibodies to the virus can confirm exposure. Most people take about 8-10 weeks to develop detectable quantities of antibodies in

the blood. Initial test may be negative even though obvious symptoms persist, procedure must be repeated in 4-6 weeks.

## 2. Antigen Test (Reverse Transcriptase Polymerase chain reaction – RT-PCR): Presence of HCV-RNA (antigen) can be detected in the blood 1-3 weeks after exposure. Antigen may be present in the blood for 6 - 10 weeks or longer depending upon host response.

Most specialists request antibody and antigen tests to understand the disease status fully and to provide better management and care.

Liver enzymes may be evaluated periodically to assess liver function. A liver biopsy may also be necessary to determine liver damage.

### Treatment:
Most hepatitis C patients in the U.S. are referred to liver specialists for expert, state of the art medical care. Before actual initiation of treatment a liver biopsy may be requested to determine extent of scarring (cirrhosis) of the liver. An effective treatment plan for specific phase (acute or chronic) of infection is devised. Interferon (alpha-, beta-, and pegylated) and rebavirin either individually or in combination are used to treat chronic HCV infection. Usually the level of care patients receive is determined by factors such as:

- Age and overall health.
- Other existing medical conditions such as HIV/AIDS and malignancy.
- Stage and severity of the disease.
- HCV type causing CLD or illness.

Patients may receive treatment for months if not years. Most prescribed medications have serious side effects such as chills, fatigue, fever, muscle/joint ache and nausea therefore patients must follow doctor's instructions and seek advice when indicated.

## HCV Prevention:

Much research is underway to develop an effective vaccine for HCV however at this time none are available. Effective post exposure prophylaxis (PEP) against HCV is also under active research. Unfortunately only limited preventive measures are available for hepatitis C patients at present.

- Transmission prevention will reduce new infections. HCV diagnosed persons are treated and immunized appropriately (for hepatitis A & B) as indicated.
- Reduce chronic liver disease and liver cancer (HCC) among HCV positive people.

## Prognosis:

People with chronic hepatitis C may develop no symptoms, suffer no liver damage, and enjoy normal living with no episodes of viral outbreaks. However people with mild or severe symptoms must take medical advice seriously. First and foremost any future damage and harm to the liver must be avoided by abstaining from alcohol, drugs, and medications that may affect liver function(s). Your physician may advise healthy ways of living that may include changing some/several habits and adopting new ones. Vaccination against hepatitis A and B may be recommended to maintain good health.

In the U.S. and elsewhere HIV/HCV co-infections are prevalent among MSM and needle sharing drug users. HIV infected persons must know that risk of acquiring HCV is much greater therefore much attention must be paid to avoid common risk factors and risky behaviors. Most STD clinics in the U.S. closely monitor HIV patients for HCV infection by periodic screening for HCV antibodies, HCV-RNA antigen, and critical liver function tests.

The greatest threat HIV/HCV infected persons face is the rapid progression of liver cirrhosis and eventual death. HIV/AIDS patients co-infected by HCV require much skilled aggressive therapy. Antiretroviral cocktail therapy may be continued to contain HIV for improved immune response. Patients are then treated for HCV for favorable outcome.

## 4. Herpes - Genital and Oral
## Herpes simplex virus – HSV 1 & HSV 2

Genital herpes is a very common sexually transmitted chronic life-long disease caused by herpes simplex virus 2. There are two types of herpes viruses: HSV- I and HSV-2. Both HSV types are uniquely different yet produce similar symptoms. HSV-I is usually associated with oral (mouth) infection causing cold sores but can also infect ano-genital area. Recurrent genital herpes with classic symptoms is caused by HSV-2. Aside from infecting genitals and mouth both types of herpes simplex viruses can infect eyes, hands (nail beds), and skin around the anorectal area. Both viruses may infect any other part of the body by scratching and itching. Group of Herpes viruses cause diseases such as chickenpox, cold sores, genital sores, mononucle-osis, and shingles.

Genital and oral herpes infections are very common worldwide - every country in every continent has this unpleasant medical problem. Millions are presumed to be infected in the U.S. alone. Many more may be infected but are not included for the count due to asymptomatic nature of the disease. It is safe to assume that herpes is the most common sexually transmitted global STD.

## Transmission:

- Herpes infection is acquired by physical con-tact with an infected person such as skin to skin contact, anal, oral, and vaginal sex.
- Infected persons can transmit HSV by body flu-ids such as blister, sore, wound exudate, saliva, semen, and vaginal secretions.
- Patients with herpes sores/blisters on the lips, mouth, genitals, and rectum can transmit HSV by intimate physical contact and sex.
- Persons who are asymptomatic for herpes can for sure infect friends, family, and sex part-ners by skin to skin contact.
- Babies and kids can acquire oral herpes result-ing in cold sores when asymptomatic adults hug and kiss the little ones.
- Many infected children may not develop cold sores and symptoms yet pass on the virus to their playmates and friends.
- Oral herpes, cause of cold sores is transmitted by saliva.

- Commercial sex workers, people who entertain multiple sex partners, alcoholics, and needle sharing drug users present high risk to non-suspecting general public.
- Women in general can easily contact herpes than men due to much larger mucosal vaginal surface that is receptive to HSV retention.
- African American women are at much higher risk to acquire genital herpes because HSV - 2 is widespread among African American men.
- HSV can be transmitted by predators of sexual assault, and physical abuse.

Children with recurring cold sores most likely are not even aware that the sores are caused by herpes. This confusing scenario places more children (as well adults) at risk. Most infected children may not develop cold sores hence will not experience recurrence of such episodes (as do adults) due to high concentration of circulating antibodies to HSV-I.

In some very rare cases people can get herpes infection of the eyes. This is usually self-inflicted. Herpes of the eyes is always caused by HSV - I. Effective treatment is available. Your ophthalmologist may prescribe cream or ointment if indicated.

HSV usually attach to the mucous membrane(s) of the host, slowly creep via nerves to the nearest ganglion and remain dormant until an opportune time to creep back to the skin surface of initial contact. This can cause full blown eruption and infection – also known as prodrome. The virus received its name herpes from the Greek word herpes (means to creep).

## HSV and Pregnancy:

Herpes (type 1 & 2) viral transmission and infection among newborns is a cause of concern. Infected mother can shed HSV during normal delivery and infect infant during passage through birth canal.

Pregnant women who acquire HSV-2 infection prior pregnancy share antibodies with the fetus. Immune mothers present no danger to the baby in the womb. But pregnant women who acquire HSV 1 and 2 during late pregnancy represent huge risk (30 -50%) to the fetus. Unborn exposed to HSV may experience mild symptoms, and in rare cases suffer extreme permanent neurological disorder and death. Some of these survived infants may also experience birth defects. Prompt treatment and care may help resolve this problem for some.

Susceptible women whose sex partners are infected by HSV 1 and 2 should be advised abstinence during third trimester as an effective means of neonatal transmission prevention. Condom use also may reduce risk for transmission to the neonate. Healthcare providers usually counsel pregnant women of late trimester to:

- Avoid oral sex with partner(s) with cold sores (HSV 1).
- Avoid vaginal penetration with partner (s) with genital herpes (HSV -2).

Infected men can reduce risk for viral transmission to their uninfected sex partners during late pregnancy by suppressive therapy. HSV -2 infected men seeking to have children should be counseled the benefits of such therapy during planned procreation process.

## Herpes Outbreak - Prodrome:

In newly infected persons the virus moves from the point of contact or mucous membrane(s) to the local nerve ending and creeps along to settle in the ganglion near the spinal cord. Virus may remain dormant or latent in the ganglia for a long time but periodically can reactivate, replicate, and creep back to the skin surface of initial contact causing skin eruption(s) resulting in painful blisters/sores. Such an eruption or outbreak is called prodrome. Prodrome may occur to people under certain conditions such as:

- Fever and flu like symptoms.
- Emotional or physical stress.
- Prolonged exposure to sun and heat.
- Certain drugs and food in some people.
- Suppression of immune system by conditions such as HIV/AIDS, malignancy, and steroid therapy.
- Unknown factors.

Most people develop sores or blisters on the skin or mucous membrane during prodromes but some may not. Such condition is considered asymptomatic. HSV can be transmitted by asymptomatic people to their contacts. Episodal periodic herpes outbreak or asymptomatic viral creeping (shedding) may continue for months or life-time for some people.

Not all people infected with herpes experience prodromes. People infected with oral and genital herpes will experience viral outbreaks and shedding at some point - but this may vary from person to person.

## Prevention of Transmission – How to Lower Risk for Genital Herpes:

Many infected men and women are asymptomatic, not aware of their infection, therefore unaware of transmitting HSV to their sex partners. Some useful tips are listed below.

- Total abstinence is the most certain way to live free of herpes.
- Prevention can be achieved by having sex only with an uninfected person who has sex only with you.
- Safe sex practices such as condom use can help but condom doesn't cover areas other than the penis. Uncovered areas such as abdomen, thighs, and scrotum can come into contact with herpes infected area and acquire infection.
- Infected persons can lower the risk for transmission by abstaining from sexual intercourse during virus outbreak (s).
- Infected persons can reduce risk for HSV transmission to their sex partners by antiviral suppressive therapy – talk to your doctor.
- Susceptible sex partners can reduce risk by suppressive therapy.
- Avoid sexual activity with needle sharing drug users, alcoholics, and commercial sex workers.
- Washing genitals, shower, douching, and urination after sex will not help  prevent herpes and other STDs.

## Symptoms:

Genital herpes (type 2) often tends to be asymptomatic and if symptoms develop, such symptoms are brief and transient. As symptoms disappear so does urgency to seek medical advice. However it is important to recognize symptoms to seek and receive prompt medical care. Absence of vivid symptoms is no guarantee of lack of infection – especially herpes. Some of the most common symptoms are:

- Flu – like symptoms such as feeling of illness, mild fever, body ache, head ache, and watery eyes.
- Mild to severe itching, tingling, or pain in the areas of outbreak - usually genitals, anus, eyes, and around the mouth (HSV-I). These initial symptoms may appear within 2 - 20 days upon exposure.
- Painful sores/blisters may soon appear at the site of infection as red patches – may persist for weeks - this can vary from person to person.
- Red patches may appear in the mouth, throat, genitals, and rectum.
- Infected fingertips become red, swollen, and intensely painful. The condition is known as herpetic whitlow.
- Uncircumcised men may find herpes sores inside the foreskin.
- Women develop painful herpes blisters/ lesions/sores on the labia, inner labia, cervix, vagina, and vulva.

- People receiving anal sex usually develop painful blisters around anal/rectal area and inside the rectum itself.
- Blisters tend to break, fuse in clusters, and may become crusted.
- Lymph nodes in the groin and neck enlarge, become tender, and painful.
- Urination can be burning and very painful due to blisters in the urethra.
- Physical activity, walking, and even moving may be painful due to lesions in the ano-rectal, genital, and groin areas.
- HSV-1 and HSV-2 produce identical symptoms - only difference is the location of sores/blisters/ulcers. Sores on the mouth/lips caused by HSV -1 are called fever blisters.
- Initial (primary) herpes outbreak can be severe, extremely painful, and prolonged than the subsequent prodromes and can cause extended illness and discomfort. Severe genital ulceration and neurologic complications may also occur.
- Sores/ulcers/lesions on skin surface such as face, neck, buttocks, pubic area, outer labia, penis, scrotum, and other areas may eventually heal (with medications) leaving annoying scars.
- Blisters on the mucosal surface such as mouth, throat, inner labia, vagina, and urethra heals clean and leaves no scabs or scars.
- Most herpes patients become used to discomfort of periodic prodromes.

- Outbreak of herpes is much more severe, intensely painful, prolonged, and frequent for HIV/AIDS persons.

## Diagnosis:

Not everyone develops classic painful and ulcerative lesions for herpes. In some people symptoms may be mild, appear briefly, and cause no discomfort or pain therefore go unnoticed. Blisters/sores in the mouth can be a result of allergies to food or medication in some people. Experienced healthcare professionals can visually differentiate sores/lesions due to allergies, STDs such as chancroid, syphilis, lymphogranuloma venereum, and herpes.

When any symptoms such as described above appear see your doctor ASAP- before symptoms disappear. This will save you much discomfort later. Any faint thoughts of just acquired herpes infection may be nerve-wrecking. Chances are you may not remember all the symptoms when you finally make that visit to your doctor's office or clinic. Therefore clearly note any/all symptoms as best you can on paper. Let your physician know exactly how you feel - itchy/tingly/fever etc. Your doctor may ask leading questions such as your most recent sexual encounter, previous contacts, previous occurrence of symptoms, location of sores and blisters. This information is helpful to accurately diagnose herpes I or 2. Additionally appropriate laboratory tests may be requested for confirmation.

### Test for Herpes I & 2
## 1. Virus Culture Test:

Herpes Viral culture test is the recommended initial procedure to confirm HSV Type I or 2 infections. Your doctor or nurse may swab the reddish blisters, place the swab (s) in culture media (tubes) for laboratory testing. Positive culture indicates viral outbreak and current infection. This test requires usually 7-10 days (if it is positive) to conclude or longer in some cases. Positive result is confirmed only if the virus is able to grow and multiply. If viral activity is not detected test is reported negative. However negative herpes culture may simply mean that no virus was present in that sample/site at that time, either because the lesion has healed (scabbed) or swabbing was unproductive. You may be asked to return for repeat test in 4-6 weeks

Herpes culture must be performed on new or just emerging blisters, lesions, or sores, and processed promptly to be accurate. Failure to grow herpes virus should not be presumed absence of infection. It may be that test is not quite sensitive therefore unreliable.

## 2. Antigen Detection Test:

Test is performed by swabbing new or aged blister (lesion or sore) and sent to the laboratory - no culture media is necessary. Procedure detects specific viral proteins or antigens for herpes (I & 2) virus. Test is not designed to distinguish between virus types but to confirm the presence of virus on the swabbed blister. Antigen test is highly sensitive yet it's not routinely available due to high cost and lingering doubts namely, negative test does not rule out latent/dormant herpes infection.

## 3. PCR (Polymerase Chain Reaction) Test:

PCR Test can be performed on exudate from blisters, lesions, or sores caused by HSV -I or 2. In the absence of symptoms, spinal fluid is the specimen of choice.

Procedure is highly sensitive, expedient, and clearly differentiates between the two types of herpes virus. This test is highly cost prohibitive and used mostly for research purposes.

## 4. Antibody Blood Test for Herpes Type - I & 2:

Most clinics, health centers, and modern clinical laboratories offer new advanced type specific and non- type-specific antibody tests for herpes. Antibodies develop in response to infection weeks or months after exposure and persist for life. Presence of antibodies confirms infection. Absence of antibodies in a symptomatic person indicates that adequate, measurable amounts of antibodies are not yet produced. Tests detect and quantify antibodies to specific protein (s) of the viral protein coat. These type specific antibodies are referred to as glycoprotein G's (gG). People infected by HSV- 1 produce protein G1 and HSV – 2, protein G2.

## 5. Western blot blood test: Available for genital herpes. Test is highly sensitive and reliable but cost prohibitive. However in situations such as sexual assault and child abuse Western blot is preferred over other tests for legal and medical expediency.

## Time to Test for Herpes:

All sexually active people especially those who entertain multiple partners and persons at high risk should periodically self-examine their genitals and mouth for unusual blisters, bumps, or sores as a precaution. If symptoms appear as listed below promptly seek medical/diagnostic help.

- Unusual sore, bump, lesion on or around ano/genital area.
- Tiny reddish painless sores on penile head or labia minora.
- Cold sores in and around mouth and lips.
- Recent sex-partner has cold sores, genital blisters or symptoms resembling genital herpes.
- People with no symptoms should periodically test for herpes and other STDs as a precaution. Occasion also presents an opportunity for face to face meeting with healthcare provider – a trusted source for information.

## Management and Treatment for Herpes:

Like AIDS, herpes has no cure (yet), but current armory of safe and effective antiviral medications listed below can treat, manage, and prevent symptoms and recurring outbreaks. The drugs don't eradicate latent HSV irrespective of prolonged systemic use. However if therapy is discontinued symptoms may recur so will the frequency and severity of prodromes.

In most people newly acquired genital herpes can cause intense pain, prolonged illness, severe genital ulceration, and neurologic discomfort. Antiviral therapy is prescribed until symptoms are resolved. Therapy may be continued for a longer period if indicated.

Established genital herpes brings on prodromes, genital lesions, and intermittent asymptomatic HSV shedding in most people. Antiviral therapy can greatly reduce pain, symptoms, and frequency of prodromes.

**Systemic antiviral drugs listed below are also useful for:**

1. **Episodic therapy:** Usually initiated immediately when symptoms appear or within days of onset of sores or lesions. Therapy relieves pain and shortens the duration of lesions due to first episodal genital herpes. Therapy is also useful for subsequent episodes.

2. **Suppressive therapy:** Reduces frequency of genital herpes outbreak and recurrence. Most persons with established HSV -2 may prefer suppressive therapy over episodal regimen. Therapy can decrease risk of transmission to sex partner (s).

    Treatment must be taken as prescribed (dosage and duration) for best outcome.

## Most frequently prescribed medications:

- Acyclovir 400mg taken orally 3 times a day for 7 - 10 days.
- Famciclovir 250mg taken orally 3 times a day for 7 - 10 days.
- Valacyclovir 1g taken orally twice a day for 7 – 10 days.

## Benefits of antiviral suppressive therapy:

- Delay in frequency or absence of genital/oral herpes prodrome.

- Some persons may still experience mild but asymptomatic outbreaks.
- Fewer outbreaks reduce risk of transmission and infection to sex partners.
- Reduce viral shedding therefore lower risk for transmission.

Greater efficiency in transmission reduction could be achieved if all three

preventive tools such as condoms, suppressive therapy, and abstinence are practiced during prodromes.

Most antiviral drugs listed above have mild to severe side effects. Intensity of pain and discomfort may vary. Some side effects can be avoided by careful attention to dosage and timing such as before or after meals. Before initiating drug therapy consult your physician and pharmacist about the side effects and ways to avoid or minimize them.

Several topical antiviral therapeutic creams, gels, and lotions are currently available. Topical microbicides in the form of compounds, gels, and creams offer pain relief and prolong frequency of prodromes when applied directly over infected areas. However an effective FDA approved topical treatment is not yet available.

## Severe Herpes and Complications:

Persons with severe HSV infection with complications require hospitalization, intravenous (IV) antiviral (acyclovir) therapy and simultaneous oral regimen.

Topical creams and gels may be prescribed to relieve pain, itching, and redness.

Untreated genital herpes can become severe with complications such as disseminated infection, hepatitis, meningoencephalitis, or pneumonitis. Patients are usually hospitalized and treated as described above. Resource for treatment guidelines is always available at: www.cdc.gov/STD/treatment/

## Prognosis:

Research is underway to improve treatment options for HSV 2. Development of an effective vaccine is a priority however we may have to wait. As in HIV, HSV life cycle from attachment to replication phase can be disrupted by various antiviral drugs and combination of drugs as described already. Currently available potent antiviral drugs can treat, prevent, and suppress symptoms (outbreaks) effectively. Viral suppressive treatment can also reduce risk of transmission.

Herpes infection is for life. However recurring pain and inconvenience can be minimized by carefully adhering to professional medical advice. A combination of antiviral drugs and topical gels or creams can suppress outbreak, reduce transmission, viral shedding, and pain.

In almost all communities in the U.S. auxiliary support services are available for HSV infected men and women. Special counseling services and treatment are integral part of HSV management. Most healthcare providers and clinics routinely encourage patients to participate in such counseling programs. Useful information can be obtained from your healthcare provider, hospital, local health department, Red Cross, private and public library.

## Visit to The Clinic or Doctor's Office:

Prepare yourself emotionally and mentally for this important visit. Request company such as your spouse, trusted friend, or someone you are totally comfortable with. A caring compassionate escort may make your trip less stressful.

Most healthcare professionals are acutely aware of their obligation to patients. They respect your privacy and put your mind at ease so relax and answer all questions truthfully. No reason to be embarrassed. If they overlooked or failed to ask, volunteer specific details so that your doctor has all the information prior to your physical examination.

Accurate information begets better care, good advice, and valuable support.

Your symptoms and location of blisters/sores/ulcers usually determine appropriate tests and procedures. At this point you may request a complete screen for STDs including HIV test. Though cost is high information is priceless and a good first step for healthy YOU.

## Coping with Genital Herpes:

Millions of people live with genital herpes for life. Some get used to the inconvenience and learn to cope but some may have great difficulty to adapt. However infected men and women can enjoy normal life but be prepared and expect the following:

- Painful, embarrassing genital sores/lesions.
- Frequent herpes outbreaks (usually 4-6 a year).
- Persons with genital herpes are at greater risk for HIV and other STDs.
- Emotional stress, mood change, worries, and concern for self and spouse.
- Pregnant women could infect the fetus.

- If herpes is triggered during labor cesarean delivery may be performed to prevent infection to the baby.
- If prodromes trigger during late pregnancy baby can suffer permanent neurological disorder, birth defects, and death in rare cases.
- For recurrent genital herpes during late pregnancy prophylactic antiviral treatment may be prescribed to avoid cesarean delivery and developmental abnormalities to the baby.

## Management of Sex Partners:

Current and previous sex partners of herpes patients can greatly benefit from physical examination, evaluation, and professional counseling for herpes and other STDs. Persons diagnosed for genital herpes must provide names of past and current sex partners to their physician so that all may receive professional care. HSV may be reportable to local and state health department in your state by law.

Your positive attitude, open mind, and willingness to open up will help you and your sex partners. A worry-free, STDs -free living is a huge reward.

Your doctor may recommend supportive services such as counseling for you and your spouse. Get all the psychological and emotional support you can for a better, happy, healthy future. Your doctor also has valuable advice to lower risk for genital herpes. Personalized suggestions may include partner selection, changes in your sexual behavior, and safe sex practices. Talk to your doctor or visit the nearest clinic if you or your sex partner(s) require periodic counseling.

# 5. Molluscum
## Molluscum contagiosum Virus Infection

Molluscum is an infection of the skin caused by Molluscum contagiosum virus, a member of poxvirus family. Infected skin develops painless, smooth, waxy, or dimpled bumps. Bumps are usually less than half an inch in diameter with a dimple in the center. Infection, also known as molluscum is very common among children and adults. Molluscum virus is contagious and can be transmitted upon skin contact. Children develop skin bumps anywhere on the body such as arms, face, neck, and abdomen. Adults usually contact molluscum by intimate sexual contact. Sexually acquired molluscum usually produces bumps or warts on the genitals, groin, and pubic area.

## Transmission:
Virus is transmitted by physical (skin) contact. Members of household, friends, and acquaintances may get infected by physical contact, sharing common items, wash towels, and other objects.

- Saliva of infected people can transmit virus to friends and family.
- Infected adults can infect sex partners.
- Physical non-sexual contact can cause molluscum among children and adults.

## Symptoms:
Molluscum warts may appear within a week after exposure in some people. It may take months for others and some may never develop such warts.

153

- Skin colored, smooth, waxy, tiny bumps appear on the skin at point of contact with infected persons' skin such as genitals, groin, lower abdomen, and pubic area.
- Tiny bumps may grow into larger bumps in some people. Usually many tiny bumps may clump together to form a cluster of warts.
- Dimple or dent in the center of bump(s) is characteristic of molluscum. When dimple is pierced (with a sterile needle/lancet) and squeezed gently, a thick whitish creamy liquid exudes that contains Molluscum contagiosum.
- Molluscum transmitted by non-sexual contact among children produces warts as above except for their location on the body. Most children develop such warts anywhere on the body but the genitals.
- Most people who develop molluscum may resolve symptoms without treatment within a few months with no scars. Immune compromised persons with skin disorders may take much longer to resolve molluscum.

## Diagnosis:

Physical appearance of bump (s) with dimple in the center is characteristic of molluscum warts. Dimple can be pierced to expel creamy core of the bump. Physical appearance of dimpled warts confirms molloscum infection from genital warts caused by papillomavirus and syphilis. No antibody or antigen blood test is recommended for routine diagnosis and confirmation of molluscum.

## Treatment:

Molluscum bumps are painless, do not itch, non- life-threatening, yet cosmetically annoying. However for many, bumps appear only to disappear within weeks or months. For restless few physician(s) may perform following procedure(s):

- Freeze the lesions/bumps with liquid nitrogen.
- Treat bumps and surrounding skin with podophyllin or trichloroacetic acid solution (TCA).

Healthcare providers usually combine above procedures to avoid scarring as a result of treatment.

Based on size, location, and number of warts, your doctor may choose to pierce dimple(s) of warts(s), dispel core, and help accelerate resolution. He/ she may train you to perform this procedure safely in the comfort of your home.

Above procedures are safe, provide comfort, and avoid ugly sight of warts on the skin. Though eventual resolution with no treatment is assured, some people prefer not to wait.

People who opt to remove warts at home need to follow physician's advice and avoid unpleasant complications and infection. Immune impaired people must opt out of "in home" treatment altogether to avoid serious co-infections. Those who opt to perform such procedure at home must follow guidelines listed below.

- Use only sterile lancets or needles.
- Wash warts and surrounding area well with soap and water. Wipe off soapy water with clean towel and then wipe with alcohol swab.

- Gently pierce dimple with lancet, turn about 30 degrees and withdraw lancet. Gently squeeze creamy core out.
- When the procedure is complete wash well with soap and water. Wipe the entire area dry with alcohol swab.
- Failure to follow procedure as described above may cause bacterial infection.
- Immune compromised persons may not be so successful in resolving molluscum. Home treatment(s) may not produce desirable results, therefore must seek expert medical advice to avoid opportunistic infections.

# PART III
## Sexually Transmitted Diseases of Bacterial Origin

## 1. Bacterial Vaginosis - BV
## Gardnerella vaginalis and Mycoplasma hominis

Bacterial Vaginosis is a common polymicrobial infection of the vagina. Millions of women worldwide are affected by this syndrome that is caused by an imbalance of vaginal flora. In the U.S. prevalence of BV is documented to be very high, may exceed 50% in the general female population. Hydrogen peroxide producing Lactobacilli are replaced by microbes such as G. vaginalis, M. hominis, and several other fastidious anaerobes producing ecological imbalance in the normal vaginal flora. Some women experience BV briefly but many continue to suffer BV for a very long time due to frequent recurrence. BV is the primary cause for vaginal discharge and malodor in most women. BV is often asymptomatic. Women at much greater risk for BV are listed below.

- Women with multiple male or female sex partners.
- Women infected with chlamydia, herpes, trichomoniasis, and yeast.
- Implantation of intrauterine device (IUD) for birth control.
- Over- douching can cause BV.

- Condom-free sex may influence the ecosystem in the vagina causing BV.
- Childbearing age women are more prone to BV.
- Women who have sex with women.
- Some women lack vaginal lactobacilli for unknown reasons.
- Sexually inactive women too can be affected.

## Transmission:

For most women BV can be self- inflicted. Condition is usually created by an imbalance of the normal vaginal flora. There is no evidence that Gardnerella, Mycoplasma, or other organisms causing BV in women is sexually transmitted by men. Treating male sex partners of women with BV has not helped prevent such episodes. By contrast women having sex with infected women can readily acquire BV. BV is not proven to be sexually transmitted but sexually associated.

Women with BV are at much greater risk to acquire STDs such as HIV, gonorrhea, chlamydia, and genital herpes.

## Prevention of Transmission – How to Lower Risk for BV:

BV as a disease is not fully understood therefore healthcare providers may not know the best approach for prevention. However a few tips below may help.

- Abstinence does not help prevent BV. BV may be self- inflicted in most women.
- Sexually active females can benefit by monogamous relationship or limiting number of sex partners.

- Proper condom use all the time can reduce risk for BV.
- Over – douching increases risk for BV.
- Physician prescribed antibiotics for BV must be taken – use all the medicine, full course as advised even after resolution of symptoms.
- Washing genitals, urinating, and douching after sex will not reduce risk.

## Symptoms:

Most women with BV are asymptomatic and some who have mild symptoms most likely ignore them. Symptoms may appear within days after intercourse, douching, or insertion of IUD. Most women with BV usually experience some or all symptoms listed below:

- Mild itching in the vagina associated with feeling of discomfort.
- White cloudy discharge that also coats vaginal walls.
- Fishy malodor. Malodor may be heavy after intercourse, douching, and during period (s).

## Diagnosis:

Pelvic examination is necessary to confirm or rule out BV. Patients may be advised not to douche but bring first morning urine specimen for microscopic examination and pH testing. Diagnosis can be complicated due to the absence of a single pathogen as in the case of some other STIs. Classic symptoms listed above obviously help suspect BV. Diagnostic tests may be performed to confirm.

- Vaginal wall/canal is swabbed for gram stain to determine relative concentration of lactobacilli.
- Vaginal culture reported as mixed bacterial growth indicates presumptive BV.
- Tests for other common STDs may be performed based on medical history and sexual activity in order to rule out BV.
- pH greater than 4.5 is considered diagnostically significant for BV.

## Treatment:

Treatment for BV requires multi-prong approach. Treatment is necessary to alleviate pain, discomfort, and reinfection. Treatment also reduces recurring BV and risk for other STDs. Total abstinence and no douching is recommended during treatment for BV. Following treatment options are available.

- Vaginal flora needs to be reestablished and rebalanced with normal habitants. Intra-vaginal lactobacillus formularies are available.
- Antibiotics may be prescribed along with topical creams.
- BV can be treated with oral or intravaginal metronidazole.
- Intravaginal metronidazole and regular condom use can suppress and prevent recurring BV.
- Women who have IUDs or cervical biopsy performed may require antibiotic treatment to prevent infection(s).
- Pregnant women are treated with creams and select antibiotics.

BV re-infections(s) are very common therefore multiple follow-up visits to the clinic may be necessary.

Lowering risk for BV also decreases risk for other STDs such as chlamydia, gonorrhea, herpes, and HIV.

Female sex partners of BV patients must be examined and treated. Most male partners do not require treatment.

Pregnant women with BV require much skilled care and treatment. Prompt attention and aggressive treatment is essential not only for mother's good health but also for well-being of the fetus. Unpleasant consequences of disregard may include:

- Premature child birth.
- Underweight newborn – usually less than 5 pounds.

## Follow – Up:

Women who resolve symptoms with full treatment require no follow – up visits.

Recurrence is common due to antibiotic resistance that may increase risk for subsequent treatment failure. This form of recurrence can be treated with different antibiotics and topical creams. For some women oral nitro-imidazole supplemented by intra-vaginal boric acid along with suppressive gel therapy has helped avoid recurrence. Several other medications are also evaluated for suppressive therapy – your healthcare provider may recommend one that is best for you.

Identification and management of sex partners has not added value nor affected resolution and recurrence of BV therefore treatment of sex partners is not recommended. However WSW must consider treatment for all sex partners.

# 2. Chancroid
# Haemophilus ducreyi

Chancroid, a sexually transmitted genital ulcer disease is not so common in North America and Europe. Incidence of chancroid has declined worldwide except sporadic outbreaks in countries of Africa, Asia, and the Caribbean. Chancroid, once rare in the U. S. has recently documented increased incidence and risk. U.S. Centers for Disease Control and Prevention (CDC) has reported 24 new episodes of chancroid in 2010 and 28 in 2009. Chancroid in uncircumcised men for reasons unknown increases risk for HIV. Therefore all uncircumcised men must be tested for HIV when diagnosed for chancroid.

Chancroid is caused by Haemophilus ducreyi, a hardy gram negative, facultative anaerobic bacterium. Infection causes painful genital ulcers known as chancroid for its clinical similarity to syphilitic chancre(s) among men and women. Men are at higher risk for chancroid than women. Uncircumcised men are at even greater risk due to bacterial retention inside foreskin.

## Transmission:

- Chancroid is transmitted through anal, genital, and oral sex.
- An infected person with or without genital lesions/sores/ulcers can transmit chancroid to sex partners.
- Unprotected sex increases risk.
- Uncircumcised men are at greater risk for chancroid.
- Chancroid, like genital herpes and syphilis increases risk for HIV.

## Prevention of Transmission:

- Most effective way to prevent chancroid is abstinence.
- Have sex with a confirmed negative partner in a truly monogamous relationship.
- New condom used the right way every time can reduce risk.
- Avoiding risky sexual behaviors such as oral/anal, genital/anal contact can lower risk.
- Cold/hot showers, washing genitals after sex, or douching will not help prevent chancroid and other common STDs.

## Symptoms:
Characteristic chancroid symptoms appear within 3-10 days after exposure. Some such symptoms are listed below.

- Lymph nodes in the groin area become tender, swollen, and painful.
- Unilateral or bilateral tender inguinal adenopathy filled with pus known as buboe may spontaneously erupt and drain.
- Tiny red bumps appear on the anus, genitals, groin, and pubic area.
- Pus-filled buboes grow in size, become itchy, painful, and eventually rupture.
- Resulting shallow ulcers may resemble herpes or syphilis (1st stage) sores, associated severe pain is characteristic for chancroid infection.
- Men usually experience more pain than women.

- For men and women urination can be intensely painful.
- Urethral discharge in men and vaginal discharge in women is also common.
- For infected men and women intercourse can be very painful.
- Infection in the mouth also produces painful sores.
- People receiving anal sex may develop painful sores in the rectum associated with bloody mucoid discharge and bleeding.

## Diagnosis:

Chancroid can be diagnosed by the symptoms described above. Appearance of ulcers/sores is an important visual diagnostic tool. Absence of herpes and syphilis with severely painful genital ulcers and tender/swollen inguinal adenopathy is also suggestive of chancroid therefore sores on the genitals need to be examined and ruled out as genital warts, herpes, or syphilis.

Exudate from genital sores or lymph node abscess can be cultured for H. ducreyi but the bacterium is not culture friendly. Following symptoms are helpful for definitive chanroid diagnosis.

- Painful shallow sores/ulcers on the genitals with inguinal adenopathy (swollen lymph nodes).
- Chancroid is confirmed by ruling out genital warts, herpes, and syphilis.
- A PCR blood test for antibodies may be requested to confirm infection.

- Yellow or bloody discharge from sores/ulcers may be swabbed for bacterial culture.
- A positive culture will confirm chancroid. Often a culture may be negative because H. ducreyi is difficult to grow therefore precautions must be taken to secure and test the specimen properly.

## Treatment:

Chancroid can be treated and cured with antibiotics. Treatment may last for 7-10 days for most patients. Severe, long-standing infections may require more time to heal therefore much more aggressive and prolonged treatment is recommended. Successful treatment also resolves symptoms and prevents transmission of H. ducreyi to sex partners. Persons with advanced disease may experience scarring of infected sites despite cure. Treatment and management plan for patients with serious complications such as HIV/AIDS, malignancies, and immune impairment may be devised according to current disease status. Uncircumcised men and HIV positive persons normally do not respond well to treatment. By contrast circumcised HIV negative men respond far better.

## Follow – Up:

Patients treated with antibiotics are usually provided follow-up care. Periodic evaluation is necessary to ensure successful therapy. Follow-up is also necessary to rule out other common STDs. This may continue for 3-6 months. If ulcers reappear exudate may have to be surgically drained and antibiotic therapy extended. It is recommended that people who have multiple sex partners be tested for other

STDs such as donovanosis, herpes, HIV, lymphogranuloma venereum, and syphilis. If initial tests for HIV and syphilis were negative (at the time chancroid was diagnosed), such tests should be repeated 3-6 months after the initial test.

## Management of Sex Partners:

Regardless of symptoms for chancroid, persons who had sexual contact with the patient preceding 10 days of diagnosis must be examined and treated with antibiotics if indicated. All persons positive for chancroid require follow-up treatment as described above. Treatment and cure also eliminates risk for transmission and new infections.

Persons treated for chancroid require supportive therapy and counseling. Risk to acquire HIV and other STDs is much greater for such patients. Healthcare providers, local health department, hospital, library, and Red-Cross are some useful resources for recovering patients.

# 3. Epididymitis
# C. trachomatis and N. gonorrhoeae

Epididymitis can be an acute or chronic infection associated with discomfort, pain and inflammation of epididymis. Severe pain in the scrotum, testicle(s), and epididymis is common. Acute epididymitis may last for less than six weeks while chronic syndrome may prolong for months. Chronic epididymitis can be differentiated into categories such as inflammatory, obstructive, or chronic epididymalgia.

Epididymitis is a sexually transmitted disease caused by chlamydia and gonorrhea among sexually active men aged < 35 years of age. For some men especially the insertive partners for anal sex acute epididymitis can be caused by Escherichia coli and Pseudomonas. In men aged more than 35 years sexual transmission is not common but can be aggravated by bladder, urethra, or prostate infection. Men with bladder dysfunction, infection, and those who undergo invasive procedure such as catheterization can develop urinary tract infection (UTI), epididymitis, or both.

## Transmission:

Sexual transmission is the most common cause of epididymitis. Chlamydia and gonorrhea, individually or together can cause epididymitis.

- Infection can be transmitted by unprotected anal, genital, or oral sex.
- Bacteria such as E. coli, Klebseilla, Proteus, and Pseudomonas may also cause acute or chronic epididymitis among men performing anal sex.
- Non-sexual transmission and infection among older or sexually inactive men is mostly through invasive procedures in the uro-genital area.
- Men of advanced age can acquire non-sexually transmitted epididymitis as a result of urinary tract infection, urogenital infection, systemic syndromes, and impaired immune disorders.

## Prevention of Transmission:

- Abstinence is the surest way to remain infection free. Have sex with confirmed infection free person who has sex only with you.

- Always practice safe sex: use new condom every time to lower risk.
- Hot/cold shower, washing genitals, and douching before/after sex neither lower risk nor prevent infection.

## Symptoms:

Symptoms for epididymitis may appear gradually or suddenly depending upon person's age, mode of transmission namely sexual or nonsexual.

- For most males epididymitis is unilateral, affects either right or left side, but rarely both sides.
- Initial host response is unilateral scrotal(testicular) pain, swelling, and redness on the infected side.
- Burning with urination, urethral discharge, and acute pain may follow.
- Sexually transmitted epididymitis can be asymptomatic in the beginning but eventually discomfort, pain, and swelling develop. Nonsexual epididymitis and testicular torsion can bring on sudden symptoms and severe pain.
- Spermatic cord is usually swollen, tender, and painful.
- Chronic infectious bilateral epididymitis is common among men who develop cysts and calcification of the epididymis caused by Mycobacterium tuberculosis.
- Men exposed to recent TB are prone to chronic tuberculous epididymitis.

## Diagnosis:

Scrotum, testicle (s), spermatic cord, and epididymis are examined for pain and swelling. Person's age, severity, and onset (sudden or gradual) of pain are important diagnostic considerations. Testicular torsion, a medical emergency among adolescents, a cause of great concern must be ruled out. Diagnostic considerations also include:

- First morning urine (if available) is tested for increased WBCs and bacteria.
- Urethral discharge is tested for chlamydia, gonorrhea, and other bacteria to rule out bladder infection.
- In the absence of profuse urethral discharge urine culture may be requested to confirm gonorrhea, chlamydia, and other pathogens.
- Presence of chlamydia and gonorrhea should be confirmed by Nucleic acid amplification test (NAATs).

Other medical conditions such as testicular cancer, testicular torsion, and infection not associated with epididymis may cause testicular swelling and redness. Physical examination and medical history may suggest testing for other STDs.

## Treatment:

Epididymitis can cause serious complications if not treated promptly - male sterility and scarring of the epididymis may occur. Prompt empiric therapy can also prevent infections such as E. coli, Klebsiella, Pseudomonas, and Proteus. Problem may be quite serious for men with compromised immune system. Men treated for sexually acquired epididymitis and their partners should be advised to abstain from all sexual activity until everyone is treated and cured.

Antibiotic therapy for acute epididymitis caused by Chlamydia and N. gonorrhoeae is initiated even before laboratory confirmation is made. The goal is to:

- Disable and eliminate infectious agent (s).
- Help patient feel better by gradually resolving symptoms (3-5 days).
- Decrease risk for serious complications.
- Avoid/reduce risk for transmission and new infections.

Several potent therapeutic antibiotics are available to treat and cure epididymitis. Antibiotics and pain medications are usually prescribed. Patients with severe pain and complications require hospitalization, complete bed rest, scrotal elevation, and increased fluid intake. Persons with mild to moderate pain are treated as out-patients. Patients may begin to feel better within 2-4 days. Fever will go away so will the swelling and pain. If significant improvement is not noticed within 48 hours physician must be promptly notified.

Immune impaired men require skilled and aggressive treatment and care for epididymitis. Men with urogenital infection, prostate cancer, and malignancies are also at higher risk to acquire opportunistic infections therefore treated aggressively.

## Follow – UP:

Patients treated for acute or chronic epididymitis must be instructed to report for a follow-up evaluation if symptoms fail to subside within 48 hours of initiation of antibiotic therapy. If swelling and pain persist periodic additional re-evaluation may be necessary to rule out serious conditions such as cancer, abscess, fungal infection, and infarction. Treatment failure is rare but is a consideration for immune compromised men.

## Management of Sex Partners:

Men treated for acute epididymitis must be instructed to identify and notify their sex partners promptly. Sex partners of infected men are presumed to be infected by chlamydia and gonorrhea if their contact with the patient was within the 60 days preceding onset of patient's symptoms. Sex partners should be treated with appropriate antibiotics. Patients are advised to abstain from all sexual activity until everyone is treated, therapy completed, and symptoms resolved. Information on prevention techniques such as safe sex practices and condom use must be stressed.

## 4. Gonorrhea
## N. gonorrhoeae

Gonorrhea, also known as clap or drip is the second most commonly reported sexually transmitted infection in the U.S. Neisseria gonorrhoeae can cause urethral infection associated with intense itching, pain, burning, and profuse discharge among men and women. In the United States alone, more than 700,000 new *gonococcal* infections are presumed to occur each year. Yet in 2010 only 309,341 new infections were reported.

The bacterium infects mucosal membranes or the inner lining of the cervix, vagina, urethra, mouth, throat, rectum, and conjunctivae of the eyes. In women, gonorrhea may also cause pelvic inflammatory disease (PID) and reproductive disorders. Men can acquire gonococcal infections of the epididymis, urethra, and prostate glands. If not treated promptly gonorrhea can cause arthritis-dermatitis syndrome and other serious complications in men and women. Infection can spread to other organs such as brain, heart valves, joints, spinal cord, and rectum. Septicemia with serious complications may follow.

Gonorrhea is a growing concern for healthcare professionals worldwide. Young, sexually active teens and adults are most susceptible not only in the United States but worldwide. Gonorrhea is very common among this age group (15 – 24) therefore risk to acquire even serious infections such as HIV, herpes, PID, and other STDs is also high.

## Transmission:

Gonorrhea is transmitted by infected persons to their sex partners. Infected persons can be asymptomatic therefore unknowingly transmit the disease. This is a true medical challenge for healthcare professionals worldwide. Better understanding of the disease, symptoms, and transmission may help overcome some of the difficulties faced by the medical community.

- Unprotected sex is the primary mode of transmission. Sexual contact may be anal, oral, or vaginal.
- Most cases of gonorrhea are acquired by vaginal or anal intercourse.
- Bacterial transmission can take place by foreplay with an infected person.
- Vaginal/urethral secretions and saliva can cause gonorrhea.
- Men and women, MSM and WSW who practice anal sex may acquire gonorrhea in the rectum resulting in proctitis.
- Oral sex can cause pharyngeal gonorrhea among men and women.
- Dirty sex toys, infected persons clothing, and wash towels can transmit gonorrhea.
- Newborns can be infected in the eyes during childbirth.
- Gonorrheal conjunctivitis in adults is self-inflicted.
- Anal/vaginal infection among children and young girls/boys can be due to child abuse.

Bacteria attach to the mucosal lining of the organs such as cervix, vagina, urethra, and mouth then make their way to the blood stream. If not treated promptly gonorrhea can lead to serious complications among men and women. Some women may not develop noticeable symptoms until infection has progressed to pelvic organs causing pelvic inflammatory disease (PID) that can cause serious conditions such as tubal scarring, ectopic pregnancy, infertility, and even death.

## Prevention of Gonorrhea – How to Lower Risk:

Strategy to prevent gonorrhea must target population and demographic areas of prevalence. Healthcare providers need to be aware of local gonorrhea epidemiology in order to provide accurate information, better care, therefore effective control and prevention. Routine gonorrhea screening of high risk people can help even more. Following groups of people are considered high risk for gonorrhea and other STDs therefore require education, counseling, and periodic screening.

- Teens and adolescents.
- Persons entertaining multiple sex partners such as college students.
- People who engage in unsafe sex or erratic condom use.
- Commercial sex workers (CSW).
- MSM are at higher risk for gonorrhea than heterosexual men.
- Ethnic minorities, persons from lower socioeconomic status (SES), and urban population.
- Alcoholics and drug users by needle injection.
- All victims and perpetrators of sexual assault and abuse.

Risk for gonorrhea exists in every demographic area of the globe. Risk factors and risky behaviors can be navigated. STD free living is possible but requires discipline and good judgment in partner selection.

## Prevention of Transmission:

- Most effective way to prevent gonorrhea is abstinence. Have sex with a confirmed uninfected person who has sex ONLY with you. Monogamous relationship can be rewarding.

- Safe sex practices and condom use can reduce risk for gonorrhea. New condom must be used every time as indicated.
- Avoid exposure to infected persons' body and genital secretions.
- Avoid using infected persons garments and wash towels.
- Avoid sex with alcoholics and needle sharing drug users.
- Avoid reusing dirty (used) sex toys and condoms.
- Cold/hot shower, washing genitals, douching, or urinating after sex will not prevent gonorrhea.
- Persons suspecting gonorrhea may request empiric/prophylactic treatment ASAP. Intramuscular (IM) or oral Penicillin within hours of exposure can prevent infection.
- Large scale screening for gonorrhea in high incidence demographic areas can bring greater awareness and help prevent some incidents.

## Symptoms:

For most people symptoms appear within 2-8 days post exposure to an infected person. Many of the symptoms are common for men and women. Due to genital anatomy risk and severity of infection for women is much greater. Some infected people may be asymptomatic (most likely women than men), but eventually they too develop symptoms.

## Symptom for Men:
Most infected men develop symptoms within 2-8 days after exposure. Most common symptoms are listed below.

- Urethral burning/pain with urination.
- Urethral opening may become reddish and swollen
- Intense irritation and itching in the penis.
- Penis may become slightly tender and swollen.
- Initial scant clear discharge may turn into thick yellow copious within days.
- Pain in the abdomen, scrotum, and testicles.
- If not treated promptly infection can lead to epididymitis.
- Intensely painful ejaculation and intercourse.
- Men who acquire infection in the anorectal area usually develop proctitis.

## Symptoms for Women:
Most women usually develop symptoms within 2-8 days upon contact. Some women may remain asymptomatic for weeks. Pain and discomfort due to complications is much severe for women than men. Women can acquire infection in the Bartholin's glands, cervix, urethra, vagina, rectum, pelvis, and upper abdomen. Infection in the eyes, mouth, and throat is also possible. Symptoms for most organs are listed below.

- Urethral burning, painful urination can persist until infection resolution.
- Bartholin's glands become swollen and irritable - intercourse can be painful.
- Profuse cervical and vaginal discharge.

- Cervical infection can ascend to internal organs such as fallopian tubes, ovaries, and uterus resulting in painful PID causing fever, acute lower abdominal pain, discharge, and bleeding.
- Some women can develop scarring and increased risk for ectopic pregnancy.
- Off and on irregular vaginal bleeding between periods.
- Risk of anorectal involvement and proctitis among women is greater due to proximity to vaginal opening.

## Men and Women who receive anal intercourse may develop symptoms such as:

- Itching, burning, and pain in the anorectal area due to proctitis.
- Rectal sores/lesions and bleeding.
- Whitish yellow rectal discharge with mucus and red blood.
- Painful bowel movements.

## Oral Sex and Gonorrhea:

Men and women who perform oral sex on infected men and women can develop throat infection accompanied by pain and strong malodor. Gonorrhea of the throat in some people can be asymptomatic for weeks.

Men and women can acquire infection of the eyes causing great discomfort, itching, red eyes, discharge, and obstructed vision.

If gonorrhea is not treated promptly, infection can spread to brain cells, heart valves, joints, spinal cord, and skin.

Pregnant women risk spontaneous abortion or premature delivery. Chances of infecting baby's eyes and throat during delivery are also real. Gynecologists welcome the new arrival with eye drops and antibiotics.

## Diagnosis:

For men, infected areas such as throat, urethra, and rectum may be swabbed for gram stain and culture.

- For most men instant diagnosis can be made from microscopic examination of penile discharge. Presence of intracellular gram-negative diplococci is considered definitive diagnosis.
- Men with symptoms in the throat, rectum, and eyes are swabbed as above for diagnosis. Most healthcare providers also opt for wet prep, NAATs or both if necessary.
- Above samples are usually sent for culture to confirm gonorrhea.
- Antibiotic sensitivity test can determine the best treatment option.

For women, diagnosis may require much more testing. Usually vaginal discharge is the specimen of choice however asymptomatic women may not have typical discharge therefore cervix is swabbed to collect pus cells. Rectum, throat, and eyes are swabbed if indicated.

- Presence of gram– negative diplococci confirms gonorrhea.
- Tests for yeast and Trichomonas may also be requested to rule out such infections.
- If instant identification is not possible, fresh swabs may be made for culture and NAATs for gonorrhea and Chlamydia. NAATs are highly sensitive and reliable.

Antibiotic sensitivity evaluation is necessary in most cases to effectively treat gonorrhea. Antibiotic resistant strains of gonococci can force therapy failure. Antibiotic sensitivity tests also suggest best therapeutic option for gonorrhea resolution.

Laboratory requires 2- 3 days to confirm presence of gonorrhea, chlamydia, or any other pathogen therefore most healthcare providers offer empiric treatment.

Some women may require a thorough pelvic examination to include or rule out other common offending microbes therefore multiple swabs and pap-smear may also be made during the initial visit.

Healthcare providers routinely test all patients for other STDs even though they were diagnosed only for gonorrhea. Persons acquiring gonorrhea are at much greater risk for other STDs such as chlamydia, herpes, syphilis, and HIV. This precaution is well worth the annoyance and expense.

## Treatment:
Gonorrhea is treated and cured with antibiotics however treatment for gonorrhea is getting to be a challenge lately due to high incidence of antibiotic resistant strains. Several

highly effective antibiotics are currently available for routine and empirical treatment. Infected adults, adolescents, and abused children may receive recommended antibiotic age appropriate regimen. Initial intramuscular dose may be supplemented by oral route. Selection of appropriate antibiotic depends upon factors such as:

- Severity and site of infection.
- Bacterial resistance to certain antibiotics.
- Patients' allergies or sensitivity to Penicillin.

If infection persists days after prescribed antibiotic therapy, a different antibiotic may be necessary for cure.

Most often people infected by gonorrhea are also co-infected by chlamydia therefore simultaneous antibiotic treatment for both is recommended.

Pharyngeal (throat) gonorrhea in most men and women can be asymptomatic and difficult to eradicate therefore requires prolonged treatment with appropriate antibiotics.

If infection has spread to blood and organs such as eyes, joints, heart, brain, and spinal cord hospitalization, intravenous therapy, and much aggressive skilled care is recommended.

## Follow - UP:

Patients who resolve uncomplicated gonorrhea within 5-10 days require no follow-up services or care. However patients who fail to resolve symptoms fully should be reevaluated for gonorrhea and chlamydia. If N. gonorrhoeae is isolated, antibiotic sensitivity is performed to select most effective antibiotic(s) for treatment.

Co-infection by chlamydia and other microbes may cause mild to severe cervicitis, urethritis, and proctitis. Repeat NAATs and culture can confirm presence of pathogen (s) which need be treated and resolved.

Recurrence of gonorrhea is common among patients who have been treated and considered cured. Most such reinfections occur due to patient's neglect and lack of understanding of the disease rather than treatment failure. Such patients require education and specific instructions to avoid reinfection. This can be achieved by repeat visits to the clinic and management of sex partners.

## Management of Sex Partners:

Prevention of reinfection and reducing new infections, a strategy if diligently followed may help most vulnerable communities fight the dual scourge of gonorrhea and chlamydia. Management of sex partners is designed to accomplish these dual goals. Therefore patients diagnosed for gonorrhea must be counseled to refer their recent sex partners for evaluation and treatment. Some patients may be reluctant to do so. Trained professionals should therefore contact sex partners of patients and explain why it's critically important to get immediate treatment and follow-up care.

Persons exposed to infected patients within the last 60 days of diagnosis should be evaluated and treated for gonorrhea and chlamydia. All such persons also need follow-up treatment and counseling. Abstinence until completion of therapy and complete resolution of symptoms should be emphasized. Benefits of safe sex practices and condom use should be explained to all patients.

Gonorrhea is a reportable disease in most states in the U.S. All healthcare providers and clinics must make such information available to local/state health department.

## Prognosis:

Early detection and prompt treatment effectively cures gonorrhea with no lingering after effects. However in rare cases some patients experience post-gonococcal urethritis that is caused by chlamydia and other opportunistic organisms therefore most healthcare providers recommend dual therapy (for gonorrhea and chlamydia) and follow-up reevaluation.

A full course of antibiotic treatment, careful selection of sex partner(s), practice of effective transmission preventive techniques, and above all safe sex can prevent gonorrhea recurrence. Most people infected with gonorrhea are prone to periodic reinfection and worse, are at much greater risk to acquire HIV, PID, and other dreadful STDs.

## 5. Granuloma Inguinale - Donovanosis Klebsiella granulomatis

Donovanosis, a chronic inflammation of genitals, is a sexually transmitted disorder caused by intracellular gram negative bacteria, Klebsiella granulomatis. Granuloma inguinale is rare in North America and most of Europe. Disease was endemic in Australia, Indian subcontinent, and Papua New Guinea but no longer. Currently donovanosis is limited to isolated populations with erratic or no health care provisions. U.S. has reported no incidence of Donovanosis since 2000.

Donovanosis is usually painless. Progressive ulcerative brown/reddish painless lesions appear on the genitals or perineum with no lymph node involvement. Prompt treatment can prevent progression of the disease and eventual resolution of symptoms. But if ignored, untreated infection can spread to bones, joints, and liver causing anemia, fever, and weight loss. Untreated donovanosis can predispose people to STDs and may significantly increase risk for HIV.

## Transmission:

Intimate sexual activity involving anal, genital, and oral contact with an infected person can cause donovanosis. Infection can be transmitted by nonsexual means, perhaps by fecal contact or ulcerative skin lesions. Infected mother can infect the newborn.

Donovanosis can be prevented by abstinence, proper use of condom, and safe sex practices.

Hot/cold shower, washing genitals, douching, and urination after sex will not prevent infection.

## Symptoms:

Symptoms can appear between 2- 12 weeks after exposure. In rare cases characteristic symptoms can appear months after initial exposure.

- Usually tiny painless, red nodules appear under genital skin or site of initial contact and slowly grow into round raised bumps.
- Sites of infection include groin, penis, scrotum, and upper thighs in men.
- Vagina, vulva, groin, and surrounding tissue can be infected in women.

- Anus, buttocks, and face may be infected in men and women - depending upon the site (s) of initial exposure.
- Eventually such bumps may grow, cover genitals, progressively ulcerate, and easily bleed.
- Infection may progress slowly for several years with cutaneous ulceration and disfiguration.
- Donovanosis is painless. No lymphadenopathy but disfiguring ulcerative lesions can be annoying.
- Ulcerative lesions can persist and grow slowly mimicking skin cancer.
- In some people subcutaneous granulomas (pseudo buboes) can appear.

If not treated ulcers heal slowly forming scar tissue around the edges, easily bleed, and can be co- infected by opportunistic organisms causing severe complications.

In some people infection can extend to pelvis, intra-abdominal organs, bones, and mouth causing anemia, fever, weakness, and severe weight loss.

## Diagnosis:

Klebsiella granulomatis is difficult to grow/culture in the laboratory. Antigen, antibody tests are also not available. Characteristic bright red ulcers on the genitals and surrounding tissue are important visual tools. Microscopic examination of the tissue specimen secured from the edges of ulcerative bump is recommended to confirm donovanosis. Presence of dark-stained donovan bodies from tissue biopsy provides definitive confirmation. Donovanosis in women can be confirmed by pap -smear test.

## Treatment:

Several effective antibiotics are available for treatment - your doctor may prescribe one that works best for you. Healing is typically slow, may require prolonged therapy for months. HIV positive patients may require much prolonged treatment.

Some patients do not respond well to single antibiotic, heal slow, and show limited progress during initial phase of therapy. Gentamycin supplemental therapy has shown favorable outcome among such patients.

## Follow – UP:

Relapse can recur 6-18 months after treatment therefore follow-up antibiotic treatment is provided until signs and symptoms of donovanosis are completely resolved.

## Management of Sex Partners:

Sex partners exposed to patients 60 days prior onset of symptoms should be examined, tested, and treated as indicated.

## 6. Lymphogranuloma Venereum - LGV
## Chlamydia trachomatis

Lymphogranuloma venereum, the most prevalent sexually transmitted disease worldwide is caused by bacterium Chlamydia trachomatis an intracellular obligate parasite. LGV is very common in tropics and subtropics. In the U.S., three most common STDs among sexually active adolescents and adults are chlamydia, herpes, and HPV. Sexually active men and women can acquire chlamydia by unprotected sex and exchange of body fluids. The bacterium can infect genitals, anorectal area among adults and eyes and respiratory system among newborns. Women can acquire infection of the cervix (cervicitis), urethra (urethritis), and rectum

(proctitis). Untreated chlamydia in women can become systemic causing severe complications such as ectopic pregnancy and PID. Men rarely experience long-term life threatening episodes. However men under 35 years of age may acquire epididymitis and MSM severe proctitis. Men who suffer severe systemic LGV can become sterile.

Rectal exposure in men (MSM) and women may also result in scarring, narrowing of the rectum, and proctocolitis.

Most infected men and women may have unilateral pain and tenderness in the inguinal lymph nodes. Some may notice tiny sores/ulcers on the genitals, the site of exposure. Pain and lesions disappear within days in most men and women therefore need to seek medical help and treatment is conveniently put off. LGV lesions if not treated promptly can cause co-infections by other sexually transmitted or non-sexually transmitted pathogens.

## Transmission:

- Infected persons can transmit LGV to sex partner(s).
- Unprotected anal, genital, and oral sex can cause LGV.
- Multiple sex partners increase risk for chlamydia.
- Commercial sex workers, college students, and sexually active teens are at much greater risk.

- LGV is most prevalent among teens and adolescents ages 15 – 24 years - the age group at greatest risk.
- MSM and WSW are at greater risk.
- Sex with alcoholics and needle sharing drug addicts can increase risk.

Though pregnant women do not transmit the bacterium to the unborn, the newborn can be infected during birth and suffer serious health problems.

Persons infected by Chlamydia are at much higher risk to acquire HIV and other common STDs.

## Prevention of Transmission – How to Lower Risk:

Sexual behavior can be an important factor in prevention and risk reduction. As pointed out already total abstinence is the surest way to live free of STDs. Have sex only with someone who is not infected and maintain life-long monogamous relationship.

Talk to your partner openly about STDs. Potential serious complications such as HIV and PID can result from untreated chlamydia.

- Avoid sex if either one of you suspect infection.
- Avoid sex with multiple partners, commercial sex workers, alcoholics, and needle sharing drug users.
- New condom used the right way every time can reduce risk.
- Hot/cold shower, washing genitals, douching, and urinating after sex will not prevent infection.

## Symptoms:

Most women infected by Chlamydia may be asymptomatic. Men on the other hand are more likely to notice symptoms early – within a day or two post exposures. For most men and women symptoms appear (if at all) within 3 - 28 days. Symptoms can appear in three distinct stages in men and women as described below.

## 1. Initial stage (First stage):

- Men may notice small, painless, fluid filled blister(s) on penile head. In women red blisters appear on the cervix, labia, or vagina.
- Blister (s) may ulcerate and quickly heal on its own without being noticed.

## 2. Second stage:

- Painful, noticeable symptoms appear anytime from 2 - 6 months after the first stage.
- Lymph gland (usually on one side) in the groin becomes tender and swollen. This is called buboe. The skin over the buboe becomes warm and red.
- Whitish yellow pus, along with red blood from lymph node(s) eruption is noticeable. Lymph nodes may eventually heal but leave ugly scars.
- Men may notice slightly swollen tender penis, scrotal pain, urethral burning, and discharge. Epididymitis may follow.
- In women cervix, urethra, and other reproductive organs may be infected resulting in severe discomfort, itching, burning pain, and vaginal discharge.

- Infection of the mouth may cause ulcers and swelling of lymph nodes in the neck.
- Anorectal exposure in men (MSM) and women can cause proctitis and proctocolitis. Mucoid/ bloody rectal discharge and painful ulcers in the rectum is common.
- Chlamydia can infect brain, eyes, liver, lungs, and other organs of the body.
- Constipation and fever may start abruptly.
- Women can suffer serious complications if not promptly treated. Painful and even fatal conditions such as ectopic pregnancy and PID can occur.
- Genital and colorectal LGV lesions can develop secondary bacterial infections or can be co-infected by variety of pathogens.

## Some common symptoms for second stage LGV for men and women:

- Chills, fever, and malaise.
- Lack of appetite, feeling of nausea, and vomiting.
- Headache, joint pain, and body ache.

If not treated promptly, ulcers may eventually heal but leave ugly scars.

## 3. Third Stage:

- Scarring and chronic genital/rectal ulcers can reappear months or years later.
- Severe scarring in the rectum can block bowel movements, cause serious complications such as proctitis, and proctocolitis.

- Obstruct lymphatic fluid flow from lymph nodes in the groin causing enlargement of genital tissue. As a result a condition known as *genital elephantiasis can develop*. This condition requires surgical intervention and repair.

## Diagnosis:

Based on symptoms and epidemiology such as genital/rectal lesions and proctocolitis LGV may be suspected. Discharge from ulcers, urethra, and lymph nodes are collected for culture, direct microscopic examination, and NAATs. NAATs (90 -95% sensitive) can confirm active infection. Chlamydia culture is less sensitive than NAATs (only 70-80%) therefore not routinely utilized. If the above procedures are reported negative antibody test must be requested to confirm LGV.

Tests for some other common STDs such as gonorrhea, herpes, HPV, HIV, and syphilis may be recommended due to increased risk.

LGV is a painful disease with severe consequences for men and women therefore it's imperative that population at greatest risk be counseled. Professional advice, much education, and greater awareness can help prevent LGV transmission. Sexually active men and women must keep the following in mind:

## Men must seek prompt medical help if:

- Penis becomes swollen and tender.
- Tiny red blisters appear on the penile head.
- Pain in the scrotum and burning during urination.
- Notice scant urethral discharge.

Slightest doubt that infection might be LGV should be a serious concern, therefore contact your healthcare provider or visit nearest STD clinic ASAP.

Women are at a greater disadvantage than men for LGV due in part serious potential consequences. Most women tend to be asymptomatic therefore unaware of already acquired LGV.

## Recommendations for Women Suspecting LGV:

- All sexually active women regardless of age must test for chlamydia at least once a year. Monogamous relationships with no history may be excluded.
- Women > 25 years of age with multiple sex partners must test more often.
- If tiny red blisters appear on the labia, vagina, or cervix call or visit your doctor ASAP.
- If symptoms appear when courting new partner visit your doctor ASAP. This precautionary measure can help avoid repeat infections and serious complications.
- All pregnant women are routinely tested for chlamydia as part of prenatal care in most states in the U.S.

Sexually active men and women owe it to each other to openly communicate about sex, STIs, and severe serious complications of STDs. Feeling safe and STD free is a tremendous gift of love.

Patients who are diagnosed for chlamydia should inform their sex partners about the disease and have them tested ASAP.

LGV infected people are at much greater risk for HIV and other serious STDs. Take your doctor's advice seriously. Test your partner and self as often as medically necessary because if your partner has chlamydia and other STDs, so do YOU.

## Treatment:

Chlamydia is treated and cured with oral antibiotics. Several effective antibiotics are currently available for LGV. It is critically important that full regimen be taken as recommended. Prompt antibiotic therapy helps prevent tissue damage and scarring. Infected pregnant women and breastfeeding mothers are usually treated with erythromycin. Some antibiotics can adversely affect the unborn and also the infant.

Rarely swollen lymph nodes (buboes) require surgical aspiration to prevent scarring and ulceration.

## Follow – Up:

All persons treated and cured should get tested 3-6 months after completion of initial therapy as part of follow-up care. Treatment failure and non-compliance need to be identified and appropriately managed with new antibiotic regimen. Patients should be closely monitored until all symptoms are completely resolved.

## Management of Sex Partners:

People who have had sexual contact with LGV infected person (s) 60 days prior to diagnosis and likely source partners should be examined, tested, and treated appropriately. If index patient is likely to entertain new partner specific instructions and guidance should be provided to lower risk.

All persons receiving treatment must be advised to abstain from sexual activity until all symptoms are completely resolved.

Management of sex partners is a confidential public healthcare service that is necessary to prevent LGV reinfections and new infections. Because many patients with LGV can be asymptomatic and some may most likely fail to recognize early symptoms, all sexually active men and women especially those who entertain multiple partners must periodically test for common STDs and chlamydia in particular.

# 7. Non - Gonococcal Urethritis and Cervicitis - NGU
## C. trachomatis, T. vaginalis, and Ureaplasma urealyticum

Non-gonococcal urethritis is yet another most common sexually transmitted infection in men and women of all ages, especially those in their teens and early twenties.

NGU is defined as urethritis caused by organisms other than N. gonorrhoeae. NGU, also known as NSU (non- specific urethritis), and post-gonococcal urethritis refer to infection that is caused by bacteria, protozoa, and virus. Organisms such as chlamydia, HSV, Ureaplasma urealyticum (formerly Mycoplasma genitalium), Trichomonas vaginalis, and yeast are most often associated with NGU. NGU is a polymicrobial infection but occasionally a single pathogen may be involved. Cervicitis/urethritis in women and urethritis in men is mostly caused by chlamydia. CDC reported 814,166 cases of NGU in the U.S. in 2010.

NGU causes inflammation, itching, pain, and urethral discharge among men and women. Cervicitis can be asymptomatic in most women but for some it can be intensely painful associated with discomfort, purulent or muco-purulent exudate, and bleeding.

## Transmission:

Unprotected sex can cause transmission of NGU. NGU in most people is asymptomatic. Totally unaware of their infection most sex partners unknowingly carry on transmission of NGU. Transmission of NGU can happen as follows:

- Unprotected anal, oral, or vaginal penetration.
- Exchange of genital fluids such as semen and vaginal secretions.
- Nonsexual transmission such as oral-genital exposure can cause NGU.
- Recurrent, persistent, and post gonococcal urethritis probably results from relapse. Rarely such episodes are due to reinfection or treatment failure.
- Pregnant women can pass on the microbes to the fetus.
- Victims of sexual assault and abuse can acquire NGU.

## Prevention of NGU:

Safe sex can prevent NGU. Prevention of transmission must be considered seriously because cervicitis and urethritis are known to facilitate other STDs, PID, and HIV. Following useful suggestions are for your consideration.

- Monogamous sexual relationship has many benefits one among them is STD free healthy sex life. Have sex only with an uninfected person who has sex only with you.
- Asymptomatic men and women can transmit infection - practice safe sex at all times. Condom use as indicated can prevent NGU.
- Oral and anal sex can cause NGU and procto-colitis.
- Avoid sex with alcoholics, needle sharing drug addicts, and commercial sex workers.
- Avoid sex with multiple sex partners and partners who entertain multiple sex partners.
- Any suspicion that your sex partner has any STD should ring an alarm! Have it ruled out by an experienced healthcare professional – play it safe at all times.
- Abstain from sex if you notice blisters/lesions on genitals. Visit your physician or nearest STD clinic at your earliest – resume sex only after treatment is complete and symptoms fully resolved.
- Hot/cold shower, washing genitals with soap and water, douching, and urination after sex will not prevent transmission of infection.

## Symptoms for Men:

Most men can be asymptomatic but some may develop symptoms for one or more organisms. Symptoms usually appear between 4 - 28 days after exposure.

- Most men who develop symptoms feel mild itching or irritation in the penis. Itching and burning can aggravate over time.
- Penis may be slightly swollen and tender.
- Burning and pain with urination and frequent urge to urinate.
- A white cloudy odorless urethral discharge may appear.
- Intense painful intercourse.
- Some men may experience far more pain than others usually due to redness and inflammation of the penile head.
- Pain and discomfort due to swelling of the epididymis and prostate.
- Chlamydial proctocolitis is common among MSM.

## Symptoms for Women:

Most women infected by chlamydia and other organisms can be asymptomatic. Some may develop symptoms between 4 - 28 days. Symptoms for Trichomonas vaginalis are immediate.

- Mild to intense itching, irritation, and discomfort in the cervix, vagina, and urethra.
- Pain and burning sensation with urination.
- Frequent urge to urinate.
- Pain in the lower abdomen due to ascending infection.
- Intensely painful intercourse.
- White to yellow cloudy odorless vaginal discharge.

Women who ignore early symptoms (all or any) as described above may suffer serious complications including Pelvic inflammatory disease (PID) that can be fatal.

## Symptoms for Men and Women:

Men and women infected during the course of anal and oral sex can develop symptoms in the anus, rectum, mouth, and throat.

- Foul odor, pus, mucous, and sharp pain in the mouth are common.
- Proctitis and proctocolitis are common among MSM and WSW. Usually red blood and whitish yellow discharge is associated with anorectal infection.

Prompt medical care and treatment is necessary – women can avoid ascending infection, severe abdominal pain, PID, and fatalities. Men can avoid epididymitis and prostatitis.

## Diagnosis:

Any/all of the above symptoms require prompt medical care. Make an appointment with your doctor/clinic as soon as possible. First morning urine sample may be requested for testing. Women may be asked not to wash genitals – douching may produce false results. Urine may be tested for white blood cells, bacteria, yeast, and Trichomonas.

For infected men with no discharge, a fine cotton tipped swab is inserted inside the urethra. Microscopic examination can detect bacteria, Trichomonas, and white blood cells. Presence of any of the above indicates urethritis.

Women require pelvic examination. A cotton tip applicator is inserted deep inside the vaginal canal to swab cervix, the sample is then examined under microscope to detect white blood cells, bacteria, yeast, and Trichomonas. Discharge from ano/rectal area, mouth, and throat are also examined as above. If test results are negative a repeat visit to the clinic after a week or ten days may be necessary. By then infection may be evident, easily detected, confirmed, and treated appropriately.

In some cases such as rape and abuse empiric treatment must be initiated.

## NGU is documented and confirmed as follows:

- Muco-purulent thin discharge from urethra.
- Gram stain of urethral discharge can detect white blood cells, and absence or presence of gonorrhea and other microbes.
- First morning specimen positive for leukocytes (white blood cells), bacteria, or Trichomonas confirms urethritis.
- NAATs for chlamydia and gonorrhea are requested when symptoms suggest infection but no microbes reported.

Based on symptoms, location, and severity physician may request tests for other STDs such as herpes, HIV, and syphilis. It is a necessary precaution one must take for good health and peace of mind.

## Treatment:
Prompt treatment is critically important to resolve NGU. Antibiotics and creams are usually prescribed. Initial treat-

ment may last for 7-10 days. Repeat office visit may be necessary until complete resolution of NGU is accomplished. NGU may recur in some people. Ignoring symptoms may cause severe complications, especially among women with persistent cervicitis. Some may be re- infected by the same microbe or a different STD therefore women require periodic reevaluation to rule out new or recurring infection. Women with unresolved cervicitis are at greater risk for serious infections such as herpes, HIV, and PID.

Men treated for NGU should be advised to abstain from sexual intercourse until symptoms are completely resolved, usually within 7 -15 days. Men with multiple sex partners can minimize risk for reinfection by abstaining from sexual intercourse until all sex partners receive appropriate treatment and complete resolution of symptoms.

## Follow – Up:

Men and women treated for NGU are usually reevaluated few days after completion of therapy. Some men may have developed complications such as prostatitis or epididymitis. Men with such conditions require specialized care. Men who successfully resolve chlamydia and gonorrhea are highly susceptible for re-infection therefore should be encouraged repeat testing in 3-6 months. Women too are required to be reevaluated for NGUs. Women with history of chlamydia and gonorrhea are at greater risk for reinfection and eventual PID. Therefore repeat testing is recommended 3-6 months after initial treatment.

## Management of Sex Partners:

All sex partners of infected men and women preceding 60 days should be identified, examined, and treated for NGU if indicated. Sex partners must be informed if chlamydia, gonorrhea, or trichomonas was identified in the index partner. To avoid reinfection patients and their sex partners should abstain from sexual intercourse until therapy is completed and infection fully resolved.

## Complications and Prognosis:
Chlamydial NGU, if not treated, may resolve on its own within 4-6 weeks in most people. However potential risks for untreated men and women are far greater. In untreated women, chlamydia may ascend to fallopian tubes, ovaries, and uterus causing infertility, severe pain, bleeding, PID, and even death. In untreated men chlamydia may cause painful swelling of the scrotum (epididymitis) and prostatitis. Yet another serious implication of NGU is one of facilitating HIV and other STDs among infected men and women.

Treatment for cervicitis caused by NGU in HIV infected women has proven to reduce HIV shedding. Reduced viral shedding lowers risk for transmission and incidence of HIV.

## 8. Syphilis
## Treponema pallidum

Syphilis, a sexually transmitted chronic systemic infection is caused by bacterium Treponema pallidum, a corkscrew shaped spirochete. Historically syphilis is one of the few recognized venereal diseases that are characterized by periods of active eruption and dormant stage (latent period) in most patients.

Syphilis infection peaked during World War II. Discovery of Penicillin (1945) substantially reduced syphilis infection worldwide. Despite best efforts syphilis represents a major global challenge with more than 12 million new infections reported every year. In the U.S., 8,533 primary and secondary stage syphilis infections were reported in 2010.

Untreated Syphilis can cause wide range of severe and irreversible damage to brain, bones, eyes, heart, skin, and spinal cord. Babies of infected mothers may die before birth and those born alive may face serious health disorders such as blindness, deafness, abnormal bone development, and mental retardation. Currently potent antibiotics are available to treat and cure syphilis. Treated and cured people can get reinfected because syphilis doesn't provide immunity.

## Transmission of Syphilis:

Infected people can transmit syphilis to their sex partners. Perception that patients with only muco-cutaneous syphilitic sores can transmit infection is not accurate. Sexual exposure to infected persons of any stage syphilis is a potential risk for acquiring the disease.

- Syphilis is transmitted by sexual intercourse.
- Syphilis can be transmitted by patients during primary, secondary, and early latent stages.
- Spirochetes require moist mucocutaneous lesions for binding, fusion, and penetration to the host.
- Touching and physical contact of infected areas can also cause infection.

- Blood, semen, and vaginal secretion of infected persons(s) can transmit syphilis.
- Pregnant women can infect the unborn, congenital syphilis has serious implications.
- Contrary to general perception blood borne, nonsexual physical contact, and accidental exposure is less common modes of spirochete transmission.

Bacteria enter the host through mucosal membranes in the mouth, anus, urethra, cervix, and vagina. Breaks and lesions in the skin also facilitate spirochete entry to host. Once inside host bacteria enter nearby lymph nodes, multiply, and quickly spread to rest of the body.

Syphilis has overlapping cycle such as primary, secondary, tertiary, and latent stages. Most patients are highly infectious (contagious) during primary and secondary phases even if asymptomatic. Disease can also be transmitted by patients of late stage syphilis with open lesions or chancre. Pregnant woman can transmit syphilis to the fetus causing congenital syphilis that may include birth defects, severe developmental abnormalities, and even death.

## Prevention of Transmission:

In the U. S. pre-marital testing for syphilis was a requirement in most states for many decades but no longer. Yet some people still voluntarily screen for syphilis antibodies as a precaution, a sure way to prevent new infection. There are other methods people can follow to protect from syphilis such as:

- Have monogamous relationship with someone who is not infected and has sex only with you.

- Always practice safe sex. New condom used every time as indicated can lower risk significantly.
- If any symptoms appear remotely resembling syphilis or any other STDs call for medical advice or better yet visit your doctor ASAP. Abstain from sex until symptoms fully resolved.
- Avoid sex with commercial sex workers, alcoholics, and needle sharing drug users.
- Avoid sex with multiple sex partners and those who entertain multiple sex partners.
- Avoid sex with strangers or persons of unknown STD history.
- Hot/cold shower, washing genitals, douching, and urinating after sex does not prevent syphilis and other STDs.

All pregnant women are tested for syphilis antibodies as part of pre-natal care in most states in the U.S. This has significantly reduced congenital syphilis and new infections.

## Symptoms:
Syphilis is a serious systemic infection that continues to inflict pain and suffering to patients in phases. Each phase has characteristic symptoms as described below.

## 1. Primary Syphilis:
In primary syphilis most people experience classic symptoms within 10-30 days after exposure. Some infected and newly infected people may take much longer to notice any symptoms and can be even asymptomatic for a long time. Most people experience severe symptoms while some may

have only mild symptoms. Some such symptoms are listed below.

- A tiny pinkish red blister/sore/ulcer appears at the site of contact. Usually vulva, vagina, or cervix for women and urethra or penile head for men.
- Usually only one blister appears but eventually more sores may develop.
- Blister soon becomes a painless sore also known as chancre. The chancre may disappear within weeks. Most people may ignore the entire episode rather than seek medical advice
- Chancres may appear on the genitals, anus, rectum, mouth, lips, and throat.
- Skin colored chancre may also develop on fingers and other parts of the body.

Prompt visit to your doctor's office/clinic must be scheduled before *blisters*/chancres disappear.

## 2. Secondary Syphilis:

In the absence of prompt diagnosis and treatment, symptoms for secondary stage syphilis appear. This may take 6 – 12 weeks (after infection) for most people and months for some. Syphilis may have already progressed to infect several organs causing variety of symptoms all over the body as documented below:

- Mild fever, headache, and flu like symptoms appear yet may go unnoticed.
- Loss of appetite, fatigue, and nausea.

- Non itching pink red patches or rash appear abruptly all over the body, especially palms and soles.
- Skin rash may quickly heal without treatment or may last for months.
- The rash can reappear weeks or months later in greater numbers.
- Blisters in the mouth and sore throat are frequent among most persons with secondary syphilis.
- Swollen lymph nodes with noticeable pain and discomfort all over the body.
- Bumpy infectious lesions appear on moist skin such as lips and anogenital area (scrotum and vulva).
- Inflammation of the eyes can result in blurred vision.
- Severe bone and joint pain.
- Inflammation of kidneys causes pain, discomfort, and protein in the urine.
- Jaundice may result in some patients due to swelling of the liver.

Secondary stage syphilis can be devastating to a patient. To avoid further complications and systemic damage, antibiotic therapy must be initiated and continued until relief is achieved.

## Latent or dormant stage syphilis:

Patients who recover from secondary stage syphilis develop latent or dormant form of the disease. In most people latent stage may last for years, decades, or lifetime with no episodes of outbreaks, recurrence, and symptoms. During early stage of latent phase infectious sores may reappear in rare cases.

## 3. Tertiary Syphilis (Late syphilis):

If a patient is not treated for primary and secondary syphilis, tertiary or late stage syphilis may result. Tertiary syphilis may be mild in some patients but may be quite severe and fatal for many. For patients of the latter category misery and suffering of a life time may be in store. Late syphilis may result in severe irreversible damage to bones, brain, eyes, heart, skin, and spinal cord resulting in bone deformities, dementia, mental disease, blindness, deafness, heart problems, and paralysis just to mention a few. Three main forms of syphilis may result in patients as a result.

1. Benign tertiary syphilis
2. Cardiovascular syphilis
3. Neuro-syphilis

The conditions just described are life threatening and fatal for most patients. Most treatment plans are also beyond utility at this point.

## Diagnosis:

Persons' symptoms, physical examination, and medical history may dictate laboratory tests for definitive diagnosis for syphilis. Dark field microscopic examination of exudate from lesion or tissue may provide conclusive results in a clinic or physicians' office. This procedure is recommended for patients with primary or secondary stage syphilis only. Most healthcare providers rely on blood tests such as:

1. VDRL - Venereal Disease Research Laboratory test.
2. RPR (Rapid Plasma Reagin) test.

VDRL and RPR antibody tests may on occasion be false due to interference. Therefor FTA is recommended to confirm initial findings.

3. FTA – ABS (Fluorescent Treponemal Antibody Absorption) test is performed to confirm or rule out syphilis. FTA –ABS is highly sensitive and specific for Treponemal antibodies. FTA-ABS test is performed on spinal fluid to confirm neuro-syphilis.

False positive test results are associated with autoimmune disorders, malignancies, advanced age, and other medical conditions. Injection drug users are also known to test positive for VDRL and RPR. Therefore syphilis is always confirmed by FTA-ABS when screening test is reported positive.

## Treatment:

Penicillin (G), the oldest of the antibiotic is still the preferred choice to treat and cure any stage syphilis. Single dose Penicillin G is injected intra-muscularly (IM) to most patients but oral form is also available. Age appropriate dosage, frequency, and duration of treatment depend on the disease stage and severity of syphilis. One dose of penicillin is adequate to treat primary, secondary, and latent stage infection. People with tertiary or late stage syphilis are normally treated over a three week period, one dose per week. Most tertiary syphilis patients may require hospitalized skilled care therefore infectious disease specialists should be consulted before initiating therapy.

Certain Penicillin preparations such as benzathine penicillin, procaine penicillin, and oral penicillin are not recommended options for all stages of syphilis. On rare occasions some people may react to penicillin with chills, fever, headache, and joint/muscle ache. Existing blisters/ chancres may even worsen. This is believed to happen to people who are at a very early stage of infection. Allergic symptoms usually disappear within 24-48 hours.

People allergic to penicillin are usually treated with doxycycline (100 mg), ceftriaxone, or tetracycline (500 mg). Pregnant women may not have this choice - they are only treated with penicillin. Treatment options just described may not be effective for people with HIV/AIDS, cancer, and malignancies. Experienced liver specialists must be consulted for much aggressive skilled care.

Victims of sexual assault and abused children are provided presumptive prophylactic treatment and follow – up care.

## Follow – Up:

Patients treated for all phases of syphilis require follow-up reevaluation and treatment if indicated. Though treatment failure is rare reinfection(s) is possible. Clinical and serologic assessment made at 6 and 12 months or sooner post treatment can be helpful to determine reinfection and patient compliance. Patients with persistent or recurring symptoms with fourfold increase in serum titer (compared with initial titer) most likely re - infected or may have failed to respond to treatment. These patients are usually retreated with Penicillin for 3 consecutive weeks - one IM dose per week, and also tested for HIV and other common STDs.

Confirmed latent syphilis is usually treated as a precaution. Treatment prevents progression of latent/dormant stage syphilis to tertiary syphilis.

HIV/AIDS patients with any stage syphilis require skilled sophisticated care by specialist(s). Periodic clinical and serologic evaluation at 6, 12, 18, and 24 months after therapy is recommended.

## Management of Sex Partners:

It is critically important that all past and current sex partners be examined, tested, and treated ASAP in order to prevent new and reinfection of syphilis. Syphilis is a reportable disease in all states in the U.S.

Patients and sex partners need counseling, treatment, and extended care and much support. Customized care outlined below should be considered:

- Patients' sex partners who were exposed 90 days preceding diagnosis of primary, secondary, and early latent syphilis should be examined and treated. Presumptive treatment must be offered to those who are asymptomatic and sero-negative as a precaution.
- Patients' sex partners exposed more than 90 days before diagnosis of any stage syphilis should be evaluated, tested, and treated as above.
- Patients' long – term sex partners of unknown history for syphilis should be examined and treated even if asymptomatic or negative for Treponemal antibodies.

- All persons who are diagnosed for any stage syphilis should be tested for HIV and retested periodically thereafter.
- Patients and their sex partners should be counseled. Benefits of treatment and abstinence must be emphacised. Sexual intercourse should be resumed only after symptoms are fully resolved for all persons involved.

## Conclusion:

Syphilis among HIV positive persons presents diagnostic and treatment nightmare. Sero-conversion for syphilis among HIV patients may be erratic and misleading. Alternative procedures such as dark field examination of lesion or tissue, biopsy of a lesion, or PCR of lesion exudate can provide definitive diagnostic information.

HIV positive patients with initial stage syphilis are considered to be at increased risk for neuro-syphilis than HIV negative counterparts. Therefore such patients require aggressive treatment and skilled follow-up therapy.

## Pregnancy and Syphilis:

Congenital Syphilis is a huge global problem. Most developed countries have made remarkable progress but underdeveloped and poor countries due to lack of resources and clear defined strategy lag behind. Congenital syphilis can be prevented by a combination of evidence based intervention. Programs must include:

- Education designed to promote awareness among pregnant and to be pregnant women.

- Mass media campaign in selected demographic areas for high risk people.
- Syphilis surveillance for public health purposes.
- Diligent monitoring, evaluation, follow-up practices for patients and sex-partners.
- Counseling concerning avoiding high risk behaviors can help.
- Instruction for condom use and safe sex practices.
- Prompt treatment, care, and management practices with emphasis on prevention of congenital syphilis and syphilis in general.

Pregnant women must be routinely tested for syphilis during initial visit to the clinic as part of prenatal testing. In the U.S. this is an integral part of prenatal care. Medical history, sex partners, and serologic testing of pregnant women should be obtained to assess risk to the fetus. Sex partner(s) of syphilis positive pregnant women must be identified and treated to prevent risk for reinfection. Pregnant women must be counseled concerning risk to the fetus and serious consequences of unprotected sex during late pregnancy. Congenital syphilis can cause:

- Premature birth
- Stillbirth
- Death of the newborn soon after birth

Survived untreated mother's child can suffer developmental problems and congenital defects. Newborn's bones, brain, ears, eyes, heart, skin, and other organs can also be affected.

## PART IV

# Sexually Transmitted Diseases of Fungal, Bacterial, and Protozoan Origin

## 1. Candidiasis - Vulvovaginal Candidiasis - VVC Candida albicans - Yeast Infection

Fungal infection of the genitals, mouth, throat, and anorectal area are very common among sexually active and inactive men and women. Vulvovaginal yeast infection is one of the most common infections women seek relief in the U.S. VVC is very common in the industrialized world and in poor countries as well. Candida species can infect cervix, vaginal mucous membrane, urethra, and anorectal area in women. Men are less likely to acquire serious yeast infections but can get candidiasis of the mouth, throat, urethra, anus, and rectum. Candidiasis is much too common among people with uncontrolled diabetes, cancer, and many other life threatening ailments including HIV/AIDS.

More women develop and experience yeast infection than men. Multiple sex partners increases risk of recurrent chronic yeast infection. Women are more likely to be asymptomatic and carriers of yeast than men. Pregnant women experience frequent episodes of yeast infection. Many other factors (listed below) predispose men and women to candidiasis.

## Risk Factors for Candidiasis:

- Persons who entertain multiple sex partners such as college students, sex workers, drug addicts, and alcoholics are at greater risk.

- Oral contraceptives promote incidence of yeast infection among women.
- Oral antibiotics kill bacteria that suppress yeast. Absence of yeast suppressing bacteria facilitates rapid yeast growth.
- Douching promotes yeast overgrowth.
- Use of spermicides can promote yeast growth in some women.
- Pregnant women are more likely to have recurrent yeast infection than non-pregnant women.
- Recurrent yeast infection under foreskin in uncircumcised men also known as balanitis is very common. Yeast cells multiply and develop a thick coating over the penile head.
- Warm, moist surface such as mouth, vagina, cervix, and urethra promotes yeast growth.
- Uncontrolled or poorly controlled diabetes can cause yeast infection in men and women.
- Immune compromised men and women are at a higher risk for recurrent systemic or localized yeast infection. Most such patients are also on multiple drug therapy and steroid supplements - conditions conducive for yeast propagation.
- Persons with low white blood cell count that may have caused by cancer, leukemia, HIV/AIDS, chemotherapy are at high risk for candidemia.
- Persons who have had invasive procedures performed such as heart valve placements, catheterization of the urinary tract, organ/tissue transplant are at greater risk for yeast infection.

## Transmission:

There is no clear consensus among experts as how yeast infection is transmitted. Most people harbor yeast in the gastrointestinal tract, genitals, mouth, and throat but rarely experience infection. Women colonize yeast in the vagina and uncircumcised men under foreskin indicating possible self-infliction. Most sexually active men and women frequently experience genital yeast infection suggesting probable sexual transmission or associated with sexual activity.

Effective transmission prevention methods may not be applicable for yeast however  safe sex practices should always be followed. Most healthcare experts agree that candidiasis is self- inflected in most patients.

## Symptoms:

Symptoms for yeast infection may vary for women and men. Affected tissue/organ may develop distinct symptoms. Most women infected by yeast rarely develop early symptoms but over time symptoms eventually appear.

## Symptoms for Women:

- Mild inflammation and redness of the vulva.
- Severe infection can cause anogenital red rash and lesions.
- Intense itching, pain, and discomfort in the anogenital area.
- Thick, curdy vaginal discharge.
- Burning pain during urination can persist until infection is resolved.
- Intense pain with intercourse.
- Strong genital malodor, much like cheese.

- Infection in the cervix can be painful, especially before and during menstruation.
- Anorectal itching, pain due to breaks in the skin associated with sparse bleeding.

Men are most likely to ignore mild symptoms altogether, however if infection is severe characteristic painful symptoms appear that are hard to ignore.

## Symptoms for Men:

- Men may notice tender slightly swollen penis.
- Penile head and scrotum may be warm and red.
- Intense itching and discomfort in the anogenital area.
- Severe pain and burning during urination.
- Men who receive anal intercourse can experience intense anorectal itch, breaks in the skin, and bleeding.
- Lesions/sores in the groin area resembling herpes may appear.
- Thick whitish yellow urethral discharge with heavy malodor.

## Symptoms for Men and Women:

- Mild fever, unpleasant feeling, and lack of appetite.
- Moderate to heavy thrush in the mouth and bad breath can persist until infection is resolved.
- Yeast infection may cause sores, severe pain, and bleeding in the mouth.

## Diagnosis:

Instant diagnosis for candidiasis is made by procedures described below:

## 1. Wet mount:

- Discharge from infected source is swabbed and placed in saline or 10% KOH solution. Yeast cells and fungal hyphae can be identified under microscope.
- If wet mount procedure is inconclusive, reddish area on the genitals or urethral discharge may be swabbed for yeast culture.

## 2. Gram stain:

- Gram stain can confirm yeast, gonorrhea, and other bacteria.
- First morning urine sample is recommended to identify yeast and rule out chlamydia and Trichomonas.

## 3. Culture for Yeast:

- Yeast can be grown in the laboratory to confirm presumptive diagnosis.

Above diagnostic tests provide instant definitive diagnosis for yeast. In some unusual cases when diagnosis cannot be made, swab (s) may be sent to laboratory for NAATs to confirm (or rule out) chlamydia, gonorrhea and other opportunistic microbes.

## Vulvovaginal Candidiasis (VVC) can be classified as:
## 1. Uncomplicated VVC - sporadic episodes.

- Sporadic or occasional/infrequent VVC.
- Mild to moderate VVC.
- VVC due to Candida albicans.
- VVC among healthy non-immune compromised women.

## 2. Complicated VVC – four or more episodes per year.

- Recurrent vulvovaginal candidiasis.
- Severe vulvovaginal candidiasis.
- Non-albicans candidiasis.
- Women with diabetes, debilitation, and impaired immune response.
- Women receiving hormone or steroid therapy.
- HIV positive immune deficient people.
- People who had multiple surgical and invasive procedures for heart, kidney, and other disorders.

## Treatment:

Yeast infections can be treated with oral medications, topical creams, and suppositories. Many such remedies can be purchased over-the-counter. If looking to buy topical creams and oral medications on your own with proper diagnosis (most preferably by your doctor) pay careful attention to special instructions on the package insert(s). Creams must be applied as directed and oral medications must be taken as per instructions for best results.

For oral therapy fluconazole 150 mg (single dose) is prescribed.

If Candidiasis is restricted to mouth, vagina, or a specific area antifungal medications are applied directly to the infected area(s) as indicated.

## Select over the counter (OTC) Intra-vaginal Medications:

- **Butoconazole** – 2% cream 5g intravaginally for 3 days.
- **Clotrimazole** – 2% cream 5g intravaginally for 3 days.
- **Miconazole** – 4% cream 5g for 3 days.
- **Miconazole** – 1,200 mg vaginal suppository, one per day.
- **Tioconazole** – 6.5% ointment 5 g single intra-vaginal application.

Prescription vaginal creams, tablets, suppositories, and oral medications are also available for vulvovaginal candidiasis. Prescribed intravaginal and oral medications must be taken as per instructions for best results.

People with diabetes, cancer, leukemia, HIV, those receiving therapy for malignancies, and other disorders affecting immune system may not respond well therefore prolonged antimycotic therapy is recommended.

Systemic yeast infection among immune impaired persons requires much aggressive skilled care. Hospitalization and intravenous therapy may be recommended for severe episodes of VVC.

Vulvovaginal candidiasis during pregnancy is treated with topical creams or suppositories. Prescribed cream(s) is applied to the infected area for a period of 7 -10 days or as directed by your doctor/pharmacist.

## Follow – UP:

Most women and some men may experience recurrence of candidiasis. Symptoms may persist or recur within months. Therefore follow-up treatment is critically important to control and cure yeast infection(s).

Follow – up visit may be scheduled 2 months after the initial visit. Efficacy of already prescribed creams and oral medications may be evaluated and changes (for better outcome) made. Patients treated for uncomplicated yeast infection are required follow-up visits only if symptoms persist or recur.

Women who suffer from complicated VVC may require prolonged simultaneous topical and oral therapy. In order to resolve VVC and keep opportunistic microbes at bay maintenance therapy may be instituted. Suppressive maintenance antifungal therapy is effective in controlling recurrence of VVC for most women but not for some for unknown reasons. Severe non-albicans (Candida glabrata) VVC is treated as complicated VVC.

## Management of Sex Partners:

Recurrence of candidiasis or vulvovaginal candidiasis (cervicitis) is not attributed to sex partners. However a few men who acquire balanitis from sexual intercourse are treated with topical creams to relieve symptoms such as dry itchy skin, breaks in the skin, pain, redness of penile head, and bleeding.

Pregnant women are prone to recurring yeast reinfection. Follow-up care and management of sex partner(s) is highly recommended to avoid such episodes.

Persons who suffer frequent recurring yeast infection are at some risk to acquire HIV however data to substantiate such claims is insufficient at this time.

## 2. Enteritis, Proctitis, and Proctocolitis Infection Caused by Mixed Flora

Enteritis, proctitis, and proctocolitis are infections of the gastrointestinal system. These common infections can be sexually transmitted, though non-sexual means are also prevalent. Different area of the intestine may be infected by different microbes. But in most patients such infections are compounded by multiple offending organisms in the same area as described below. Infection(s) can be severe and even fatal in immune impaired persons.

## A. Enteritis
## Giardia lamblia

Enteritis is an infection and inflammation of the small intestine caused by Giardia lamblia, a single celled parasite. Giardia can cause abdominal cramps, pain, and diarrhea. Parasite is usually found in human feces of infected and healthy people.

Enteritis is ubiquitous - no country in the world, rich or poor is exempt. But the disease is most common among children living in poor under developed countries with much desirable sanitary conditions. In the U.S. too, enteritis is one of the most common parasitic infection of the gastrointestinal system. Nonsexual mode of transmission of Giardia is very common but sexual transmission is the focus of this guide.

### Figure 6
### Giardia lamblia

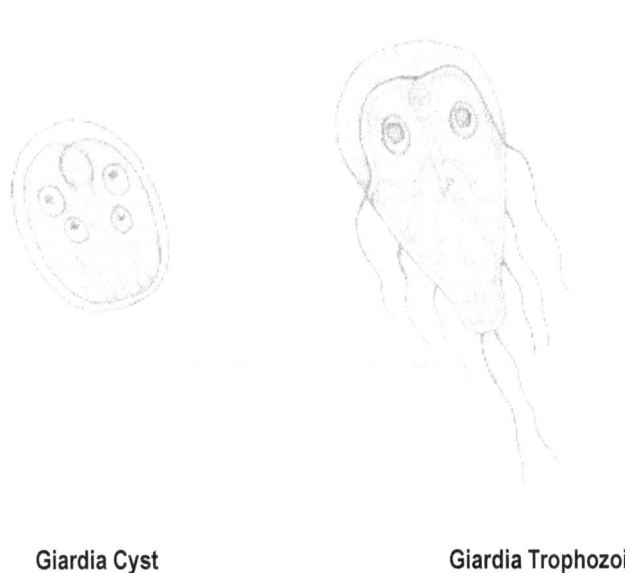

Giardia Cyst        Giardia Trophozoite

## People at Risk:

- Persons whose sexual practices involve oral – anal contact are at greater risk to acquire Giardia lamblia.
- Giardia infection is common among homosexual men and women.
- Persons who have low stomach acidity, had their stomach removed surgically, have chronic pancreatitis, or have impaired immune system can acquire enteritis by non-sexual route.

- Immune impaired people with disorders such as leukemia, cancer, and HIV/AIDS can acquire enteritis by opportunistic organisms such as CMV, Cryptosporidium, Isospora, and Microsporidium, Mycobacterium avium complex (MAC), Campylobacter, Salmonella, and Shigella.
- People visiting third world countries such as Asia, Africa, South America, and the Caribbean may acquire Giardia from water and food.
- People living in slums, crowded, unsanitary surroundings, institutional environments are at greater risk for enteritis.

## Transmission:

- Oral /anal contact increases risk for Giardia.
- Transmission and acquisition of Giardia is most likely sexually associated rather than sexually transmitted in most people.
- Improperly cooked food, unwashed fruit, and vegetables can cause enteritis by non-sexual means.
- Children can pass giardia cysts to their classmates, playmates, and adults by sharing food and water.
- People living in crowded surroundings as described above can acquire enteritis by sharing food, drinks, and lack of sanitation.

Flagellated giardia also known as trophozoite infects intestinal walls. Giardia produces tiny cysts that are excreted with feces. Persons consume contaminated food and water containing cysts. Ingested cysts localize in the new host's small intestine, hatch to produce infectious trophozoites causing enteritis. Protozoan life cycle repeats continuously producing more trophozoites and many more cysts to infect new host.

## Prevention of Enteritis:

Safe sex practices can prevent transmission of enteritis therefore patients must be counseled to change/modify sexual behavior. Safety of food, snacks, and water must be preserved. General public, especially immune compromised persons must follow safe food preparation and consumption practices listed below.

## How to Prevent Giardia Infection:

- Safe sexual practices avoiding oral/anal contact.
- Consume properly cooked food – use thermometer to assure food safety.
- Consume only thoroughly washed fruit and vegetables. Tubers such as beets, carrots, potatoes, sweet potatoes, turnips, and radish must be peeled and washed.
- Utensils, plates, and glassware must be washed in the dishwasher with hot water cycle.
- Wash hands with soap and warm water before and after visiting rest rooms.
- People handling and cooking food must thoroughly wash hands.

## Symptoms:

Symptoms for sexual or non-sexual enteritis are usually mild for most people but can be severe for immune compromised persons.

- Chills, mild fever, and malaise.
- Abdominal cramps and pain due to swelling of the intestine.
- Lack of appetite, nausea, and vomiting.
- Excessive belching and increased gas.
- Diarrhea with bloody mucous and rectal discharge.
- Some people may experience rapid weight loss.

## Diagnosis:

Symptoms described above may be suggestive of enteritis. However a definitive diagnosis can be made by examining multiple stool samples. Giardia lamblia trophozoites and cysts can be identified under microscope and confirmed by culture if necessary. Bacterial culture for organisms such as campylobacter, salmonella, and shigella may be requested for HIV suspected and immune impaired people. Some HIV/AIDS patients may require tests for opportunistic microbes also.

## Treatment:

Several potent drugs are available to resolve enteritis caused by Giardia. Metronidazole is often prescribed because it has shown fewer side effects in most people. Bacterial co - infection is treated with appropriate antibiotics. Prompt treatment for the kind of infection at hand may save much inconvenience and discomfort. It's critically important that medications be taken as prescribed. Enteritis caused by non-sexual means such as poor hygiene, improper food handling, and inadequate washing also requires prompt medical care. Members of infected family are examined and treated as a precaution.

## Follow-up:
New enteritis infection and reinfection is difficult to distinguish. Some patients may also experience treatment failure therefore follow-up visit to doctor/clinic is necessary. Evaluation, counseling, and change of medication may be appropriate.

## Management of Sex Partners:
If enteritis was a result of sexual activity patient's sex partner(s) need to be evaluated and treated accordingly. Patients are encouraged to reach out for partners and recommend treatment ASAP. Patient and sex partners are counseled abstinence until symptoms are resolved fully.

## B. Proctitis
## Infection by Mixed Flora

Proctitis is an infection and inflammation of the mucosal lining of the rectum. Infection can cause severe anorectal pain and bloody discharge. Multiple pathogens such as N. gonorrhoeae, chlamydia, Treponema, and HSV, individually or as mixed flora can cause sexually transmitted proctitis. Acute proctitis is common among persons receiving anal sex. Proctitis in HIV positive persons caused by HSV can be very severe and painful.

## Proctitis can be also caused by non-sexual means such as:

- People with Crohn's disease or ulcerative colitis.
- Radiation therapy for rectum or around the rectum.
- Salmonella and opportunistic bacteria can cause proctitis among persons receiving antibiotic therapy.

## Transmission:

- Infected person can transmit pathogens by anal penetration in men and women.
- Proctitis is very common among MSM and WSW.
- Women with genital infection can self- infect due to proximity to anorectal area.
- Sex toys or foreign objects can cause damage and infect mucosal lining of the rectum causing acute proctitis.

## Prevention of Proctitis:

- Transmission of infection can be prevented by changing/modifying sexual behavior that cause proctitis.
- Safe sex practices such as condom used every time the right way can help.
- Women with genital infection must carefully avoid anorectal exposure to genital discharge.
- MSM and WSW must use barriers as preventive tools.

- Avoid insertion of unsafe foreign objects into the rectum.

## Symptoms:

Symptoms for proctitis are usually pathogen (s) dependent. Mild to severe symptoms may appear within days of exposure.

- Itching, pain, and discomfort in the anorectal area.
- Urge for non- productive bowel movement and feeling of constipation.
- Bloody mucoid discharge from anorectal area.
- Proctitis caused by gonorrhea can be intensely painful with affluent anorectal bloody discharge.
- Proctitis caused by herpes and syphilis may produce painful lesions in the rectum.
- Proctitis in HIV/AIDS patients can be extremely harsh, severe, and even fatal.
- Radiation therapy in or around rectum may also cause symptoms of proctitis but not the disease.

## Diagnosis:

Diagnosis of proctitis requires careful evaluation of symptoms. Procedures may include anoscopy, proctoscopy, or sigmoidoscopy but proctoscopy is the procedure of choice to evaluate anorectal lining. Lesions in the mucosal wall indicate infection.

Multiple stool samples may be required for microscopic examination and culture. Identification of bacteria can determine cause of proctitis: sexual or non-sexual.

Rectal discharge may be examined for white blood cells, parasites, and bacteria.

- Pathogen(s) identification and confirmation can be made by culture.
- If herpes or syphilis lesions are present blood tests must be performed to confirm.
- Additional tests and procedures may be necessary to determine the cause of proctitis among immune impaired persons.

## Treatment:

Treatment plan for proctitis is developed based on the infectious agent(s).

- Antibiotics are prescribed to cure specific bacterial proctitis.
- Metronidazole or vancomycin may be prescribed when normal intestinal flora must be replaced. Appropriate medication(s) are also prescribed to relieve pain.
- Laboratory results may suggest additional or different pathogens than originally presumed. Appropriate medication (s) must be selected.
- Proctitis caused by HSV/syphilis requires skilled specialized care.

## Follow - Up:

Follow-up visit to the clinic may be necessary to avoid reinfection, new infection, and treatment failure though reinfection might be difficult to distinguish from treatment failure. Patients are reevaluated 2-4 weeks after initial treatment. Different antibiotic may be prescribed based on severity of symptoms or microbial resistance.

## Management of Sex Partners:

Patients' sex-partners should be identified, evaluated and treated for proctitis. Management of sex partner(s) is critical to prevent reinfection and new episodes. Sex partners should be evaluated for any disease diagnosed in the index patient and treated with appropriate medications. Patient and sex partners should be counseled abstinence until symptoms resolved fully.

## C. Proctocolitis
## Infection by Mixed Flora

Proctocolitis, yet another gastrointestinal disorder affects colon and rectum, causing intense pain, bleeding, bloody mucosal discharge, and diarrhea. Infection and inflammation of colon and rectum can be very painful. Proctocolitis is common among sexually active MSM and women with multiple sex partners.

Men and women with this disorder are usually infected by one or more microbes listed below:

- Bacteria such as campylobacter, salmonella, and shigella.
- Chlamydia, the ubiquitous infectious agent.
- Entamoeba histolytica - a protozoan.
- Most organisms causing enteritis and proctitis are suspect for proctocolitis.

## Transmission:

- Infected person can transmit proctocolitis by anal/oral or oral/genital sex.

- Women can self- infect as in proctitis.
- MSM and WSW are at greater risk.
- Sharing unsafe, dirty sex toys can cause procto-colitis.
- Sharing food, beverages, and clothing with infected persons may also cause infection.

## Prevention of Proctocolitis:

- Risk for enteritis, proctitis, and proctocolitis can be reduced by safe sex and good hygiene practices.
- Risky sexual behaviors must be avoided.
- Thoroughly wash hands with soap and water before and after visits to the rest room.
- Avoid sharing clothes worn by infected people as a precaution.
- Consume well cooked meals, and thoroughly washed fruits, and veggies.

## Symptoms:

Symptoms for proctocolitis usually depend upon the specific offending microbe. Most symptoms for proctocolitis and proctitis are similar.

- Severe abdominal cramps and pain within days of exposure.
- Diarrhea follows soon after, watery stool with mucous and blood.
- Entamoeba infection may produce fever, intermittent diarrhea, and gas.
- Bloating and stomach upset are common.

- Intense pain, burning, and itching in the anorectal area.

Immune impaired patients may experience severe symptoms and intense pain. Campylobacter, shigella, chlamydia, cytomegalovirus (CMV), Entamoeba histolytica, HSV, syphilis, and HIV can complicate diagnosis and treatment.

## Diagnosis:

Diagnostic procedures as described for proctitis may also be performed. Infected areas of the colon and rectum may be examined by a sigmoidoscope or colonoscope. Tissue samples along with swab(s) for mucous discharge may be obtained during this examination.

Stool samples may be requested for microscopic examination and culture for entamoeba, giardia, and bacteria. Laboratory tests are performed to determine the cause of infection (bacteria, entamoeba, giardia, or virus). Among persons with HIV/AIDS, several other infectious agents and opportunistic microbes may be present.

## Treatment:

Microbes not involved with infection are carefully excluded and medication(s) prescribed to counter pathogen (s) causing proctocolitis.

- Salmonella, shigella, and other bacteria are treated with appropriate antibiotics.
- Appropriate medications for entamoeba and giardia may be prescribed.

- If viral involvement is confirmed suppressive therapy may be initiated. Management of viral infection may require much skilled care and consultation with specialists.

## Follow – Up:

Periodic follow-up visits to the clinic/physician are necessary in order to remedy and resolve infection fully. Certain infectious agents described above require aggressive and prolonged treatment. Reinfection and treatment failure issues are a concern and should be avoided for complete recovery.

HIV positive and immune impaired persons require much skilled specialized care.

## Management of Sex Partners:

Patient's sex partners should be identified, examined, and evaluated for any of the gastrointestinal diseases diagnosed in the index patient and treated as per guidelines. Treatment must be continued until patient and partners are cured and symptoms resolved fully. Patient and partners should be counseled abstinence and avoid suspect sexual behavior until everyone is symptom free.

## 3. Pelvic Inflammatory Disease - PID
## Chlamydia, Gonorrhoeae, and Mixed Vaginal Flora

Pelvic inflammatory disease is a serious complication of STDs affecting upper genital organs among women. Reproductive organs such as fallopian tubes, ovaries, and uterus can be infected by one or more pathogens. In most women pelvic peritoneum, the lining of the pelvic organs, and abdomen also acquire infection. This serious inflammatory painful disorder may include any combination of endometritis, salpingitis, tubo-ovarian abscess, and pelvic peritonitis. Women who acquire PID are at high risk for even serious conditions such as:

- Ectopic pregnancy
- Tubal infertility
- High risk for fatality

Women infected by chlamydia, gonorrhea, and some other STDs receiving delayed treatment or no treatment at all are at much greater risk for serious complications. Besides chlamydia and gonorrhoeae, gardnerella, mycoplasma, and several other microbes comprising vaginal or opportunistic flora may cause life threatening PID.

PID is common all over the world. PID is not reportable therefore data is sketchy and exact figures and prevalence are unknown. In the U.S., an estimated one million PID episodes are identified but the number is believed to be much higher. Timely intervention, treatment, and care can significantly reduce risk and fatalities.

## Women who are at Risk for PID:

- Sexually active women of childbearing age
  15 -25 are at much higher risk. Risk for PID is
  relatively low for women aged > 35 years.
- Women who had first intercourse at young age
  such as 18 years or younger.

- Women who entertain multiple and concurrent sex partners.
- Women younger than 25 years of age who practice unsafe sex are at greater risk than older counterparts.
- Women with IUD implant.
- Women who have abortion(s) performed are at great risk. If the procedure was performed by a non-professional the risk is much greater.
- Women who have invasive gynecological procedure(s) performed.
- Over-douching can increase risk for PID.

## Transmission:

- PID is a complication of one or more episodes of STI. Sexual contact with persons with any STD can cause genital infection leading to PID.
- Untreated or even asymptomatic STDs can eventually ascend to upper reproductive organs causing PID.
- Excessive douching can cause imbalance of vaginal flora. Depletion of normal vaginal bacteria such as Lactobacilli can facilitate PID.
- Using or sharing "dirty unsafe" sex-toys can cause vaginal infection.
- For unknown reasons women who smoke and use drugs are at higher risk for PID.
- Some women may acquire PID upon IUD, abortion(s), and other exploratory or corrective invasive gynecological procedures.

- For most women, risk for PID is much higher during their menstrual cycle.

## Tips for Women to Lower Risk for PID:

- Avoid STD/PID. Have sex only with someone who is free of any STD and has sex only with you in a monogamous relationship.
- Avoiding any STD will prevent PID. Communicate with your (to be) sex partner. Avoid sex if genitals have any unusual sores, bumps, or lesions.
- Routine screening and treatment for chlamydia, gonorrhea, BV, and other STDs among sexually active women can lower risk for PID.
- Condoms used as indicated every time may reduce risk for some STDs but not all.
- Substance abuse, alcohol, and smoking can increase risk for STIs and PID.
- Periodic genital self-examination, especially after sexual encounter for unusual itch/rash/ discharge can help detect STDs early therefore prompt medical treatment.
- Douching, urinating, and washing after sex will not prevent STDs and PID.
- Discuss safe sex procedures with your doctor and practice them with your partner.

## Symptoms:
PID can be asymptomatic for many women. In some women PID can cause mild symptoms and for some the symptoms may be very severe.

Symptoms may appear any time after an episode of STI or menstrual period. In some women symptoms may appear gradually - months after STI. Some may notice symptoms abruptly - most likely result of an asymptomatic infection that was never treated. Most symptoms listed below may or may not be common for all and may not appear in the order described.

- Mild pain in the lower abdomen and pelvis may turn into chronic and persistent.
- Pain may appear on one side or both. Pain may spread abruptly to internal genital organs.
- Chills and mild fever accompanied by nausea and vomiting. High fever and moderate to severe symptoms may follow.
- Irregular bleeding during and between periods and moderate to heavy vaginal discharge with malodor.
- Some women may notice thick whitish discharge with malodor, sign of gonorrhea involvement.
- Intense pain and burning during urination.
- Painful intercourse.

## Medical Examination for PID:

If any of the above symptoms appear post sexual experience or menstruation call your doctor for an immediate appointment. Also consider some other reasons listed below to request urgent medical advice.

- Intense painful intercourse.
- Light or heavy vaginal discharge with malodor.

- Intermittent bleeding between periods.
- Your sex partner has chlamydia, gonorrhea, or other STD.
- Your sex partner has symptoms for any STD such as burning, itching, pain, or an unusual discharge.

## Diagnosis:

PID can be misdiagnosed for other gynecologic, gastrointestinal, and urogenital disorders. There is no gold standard nor minimal criteria for precise diagnosis therefore women with symptoms described above must patiently explain and provide information such as onset, organ(s) affected such as lower abdomen, urethra, vagina, and severity of such symptoms. Gynecological, obstetric, medical, sexual, and social history may also be factors helpful for definitive diagnosis of PID. PID is a very serious infection with life threatening consequences. Slightest discomfort in the pelvis or lower abdomen days or weeks after intercourse may be due to PID. Women who have any of the above symptoms must see a doctor ASAP. Prompt diagnosis expedites treatment and cure.

A thorough pelvic examination and multiple gynecological procedures listed below may be performed based on information you provide.

- Pelvic examination to determine tenderness of the cervix, uterus, and other organs.
- Pap-smear, swab(s) for microscopic examination, and bacterial culture.
- Vaginal fluid/secretion screened for leukocytes (WBCs).

- Sensitive NAATs for chlamydia and gonorrhea may indicate PID.
- Your physician may perform laparoscopy and an ultrasound to confirm PID. Procedures help determine (visually and physically) damage to fallopian tubes and presence of abscess in the internal genitals.
- Endometrial biopsy to confirm/rule out endometritis.
- Blood tests for elevated WBC, sedimentation rate (Sed-rate), and C-reactive protein.

Most STDs are confirmed on the basis of minimum criteria but for PID such golden rule is just not available therefore several visits to the clinic and more sophisticated diagnostic procedures may be necessary. If symptoms still persist following specific diagnostic procedures may be recommended.

1. **Endometrial biopsy** for histopathology and evidence of endometritis.
2. **Laparoscopy** to determine abnormalities consistent with PID.
3. **Trans-vaginal MRI** (Magnetic Resonance Imaging), sonography, or Doppler Studies may indicate inflammation and infection suggesting PID.

## Treatment:
Antibiotics, creams, and other medications are available to treat and cure PID. When definitive diagnosis cannot be made empiric broad spectrum antibiotic treatment may be

initiated. Your physician may also prescribe antibiotics based on your risk for STDs and PID.

Treatment is usually initiated as soon as presumptive diagnosis has been made to prevent long term damage to patient's health. Treatment must consist of antibiotics to fight chlamydia, gonorrhea, BV, and other common STDs. If anaerobes or opportunistic organisms are suspected antibiotic regimen should be changed accordingly.

In some severe cases of PID much more aggressive treatment may be necessary which may include bed rest, hospitalization, and intravenous administration of antibiotics.

Pregnant women who are suspected acquiring PID are usually hospitalized for much aggressive skilled care and antibiotic therapy. This precaution is necessary to avoid maternal morbidity, complications, and problems during child birth.

## Consequences of NO Medical Treatment and Care:

Women who have PID and get no treatment are in for severe short term (death) and long term consequences such as:

- Scarring of internal reproductive organs such as uterus, fallopian tubes, and others.
- Persistent chronic pain in the pelvis and lower abdomen.
- Infertility - women who delay treatment for PID or suffer recurrence of PID are most unlikely to conceive.
- Women who conceive most likely have an ectopic pregnancy. In an ectopic pregnancy

fertilized egg grows inside the fallopian tube(s). This can cause severe pain, fallopian tube rupture, heavy internal bleeding, and death.

## Follow – Up:

Initial treatment with appropriate antibiotics usually improves pain, tenderness, and relieves symptoms. Patients who do not respond within 72-96 hours require additional diagnostic procedures upon immediate hospitalization. Surgical intervention may be necessary.

Antimicrobial regimen assessment may determine treatment failure or inappropriate prescription. Most women with chlamydia and gonorrhea are known to have high reinfection rate within 6 months of treatment. Repeat testing is offered to such patients 3-6 months after initial treatment. As a precautionary measure women diagnosed with acute PID are screened for HIV.

## Management of Sex Partners:

Management of sex partners is critically important to avoid reinfection therefore all past and current male sex partners of women with PID should be examined and treated if they had sexual contact with the patient 60 days prior onset of symptoms. Many males infected with chlamydia and gonorrhea can be asymptomatic therefore empirical therapy is offered to prevent recurrence of STD and PID.

Patients and sex partners should follow up with periodic visits to the clinic or doctor and abstain from sexual intercourse until all are symptom free.

HIV positive women may not respond predictably to treatment and therapy like their HIV negative counterparts.

Most HIV infected women with PID are at higher risk of acquiring opportunistic infections from variety of otherwise non-pathogens.

## Prognosis:

PID is a huge concern for young sexually active and pregnant women. PID prevention and strategy for risk reduction requires serious consideration and extra-ordinary effort. PID can be prevented (for many women) and risk lowered significantly for many more by steps listed below:

- Sexually active women should avoid risks for any STIs.
- Avoid sex with multiple partners and persons entertaining multiple partners.
- Avoid sex with alcoholics and needle sharing drug users.
- Avoid sex with strangers and persons of unknown medical history.
- Sexually active women should periodically screen for chlamydia and gonorrhea.
- Sexually active and not so active women should periodically screen for STDs including HIV.
- Sexually active, not so active and childbearing age women should periodically examine their genitals for lesions, sores, or bumps preferably within days after intercourse. Even painless lesions must not be ignored.
- Prompt diagnosis and treatment can produce favorable outcome.

# 4. Trichomoniasis
## Trichomonas vaginalis

Trichomoniasis, a very common sexually transmitted disease of the vagina, vaginal canal, and urogenital tract is caused by a single celled flagellated protozoan parasite Trichomonas vaginalis. Trichomoniasis is more prevalent among women than men. Women aged more than 30 years are at much greater risk for vaginitis caused by Trichomonas. Such risk is much higher for African American women than to women of other ethnic groups. In men, Trichomonas can infect bladder, prostate, and urethra. Over 3 million cases of trichomoniasis are reported in the U.S. annually.

Most men infected with Trichomonas are asymptomatic, often seek no medical advice, yet can actively transmit infection to their sex partners. Men with any mild symptoms such as slight burning and itch ignore them altogether. Women usually experience intense vaginal/vulvar itching accompanied by diffuse vaginal discharge and much discomfort. Trichomoniasis is very common among commercial sex workers and intravenous drug users.

## Transmission:
Trichomonas is transmitted by sexual intercourse.

- Women can acquire Trichomonas from infected men or women.
- Men can get it only from infected women.
- Women who have multiple sex partners and history of STDs are at much higher risk for trichomoniasis.

- Most drug users and alcoholics are known source for trichomoniasis.
- Most commercial sex workers are a steady source for Trichomonas infection.
- Mother can infect baby during normal child-birth. Newborns' genitals and lungs may be affected.

## How to Lower Risk for Trichomoniasis:

Trichomoniasis can be prevented by avoiding/lowering risk as described below.

- Abstinence is the surest way.
- Monogamous relationship and sex only with infection free person can help.
- Condoms can lower risk if used the right way every time.
- Avoid sex with commercial sex workers.
- Avoid sex with multiple partners and partners with multiple sex partners.
- Avoid sex with alcoholics, drug users, and strangers of unknown medical history.
- Hot/cold shower, washing genitals, douch-ing, and urinating after sex will not prevent or lower risk.

Dysuria and opaque discharge are signs of impending infection. Avoid sex and seek prompt medical treatment to relieve symptoms. Resume sexual activity only when symp-toms resolved fully.

## Symptoms:

Symptoms for trichomoniasis appear about 4-28 days after exposure. Symptoms in men and women may be different.

## Symptoms for Women:

- Irritation and intense itching of the vagina and labia.
- Redness and inflammation of the vulva.
- Yellow greenish discharge from vagina with fishy malodor.
- Lymph nodes in the groin become tender and swollen.
- Pain and burning during urination.
- Urge of frequent urination.
- Intercourse may be acutely painful.

## Symptoms for Men:

Men also experience a degree of discomfort however most men may be asymptomatic and some may have mild symptoms that are conveniently disregarded. But some may experience all or some of the symptoms listed below.

- White yellowish discharge from the urethra.
- Mild itching of the penis and urge for frequent urination.
- Pain and burning during urination.
- Slight pain and irritation in the scrotum and prostate.
- Intercourse and ejaculation may be intensely painful.

## Diagnosis:

Microscopic examination of vaginal secretion or wet prep can be performed in a clinic/laboratory for fast results. Trichomonas can be identified by its characteristic flagellar movement under bright light.

- First morning urine sample may also provide prompt results. Concentrated urine is ideal for visual identification of Trichomonas.
- When visual tests fail to confirm trichomoniasis vaginal discharge/swabs may be secured for NAATs. Sensitivity for NAATs is 85-98%.
- Reliable and highly sensitive Trichomonas culture is recommended for definitive diagnosis.

Patient's male sex partners seek treatment rather than cost prohibitive diagnostic tests. Men whose sex partner(s) suffer recurrent trichomoniasis are most likely the active transmitters but asymptomatic.

## Treatment:

Single dose oral regimens such as metronidazole and tinidazole are available to treat and cure trichomoniasis. Dose and duration may vary for patients with previous history or resistance to medication. Metronidazole resistant Trichomonas can be treated with tinidazole. Prescribed oral medication should be taken as instructed. If first course fails to cure and resolve symptoms fully, second and third course may be necessary. If drug resistance is the reason for treatment failure alternate medication should be prescribed.

Cream and ointments do not eliminate infection in the urethra and genitals but only relieve symptoms.

Pregnant women need to be alarmed if infected by Trichomonas. Medications may adversely affect baby's health therefore physician must be informed so appropriate medication may be prescribed.

Untreated trichomoniasis can cause complications for men and women, especially pregnant women. Some are listed below.

## Men:

- Untreated trichomoniasis in men may lead to bladder, prostate, and scrotal (Epididymitis) infection.
- Untreated asymptomatic men may serve as source for sex partner's infection and reinfection.

## Women:

- Untreated trichomoniasis in women may increase risk for HIV and PID.
- Pregnant women are most likely to give birth to premature underweight babies.
- Infant may acquire genital or respiratory trichomoniasis.

Infected men and women must take precautions to protect themselves. A few useful suggestions listed below can help.

- Testing for common STDs must be considered during the initial visit to the clinic.
- Ttrichomoniasis infection and re-infection can be prevented by safe sex practices.
- Avoid sex if symptoms appear but contact your healthcare provider ASAP.
- If symptoms appear no matter how faint call your physician ASAP – prompt treatment can save much inconvenience and pain.

## Follow – Up:

Some women, for unknown reasons are prone to reinfection within months after initial treatment - most men rarely suffer reinfection. Follow – up visit for women at high risk should be scheduled for reevaluation. Reinfection can be attributed to untreated sex partner, treatment failure, or drug resistance. Careful evaluation may determine corrective measures. Alternative medication such as tinidazole or a higher dose of metronidazole may be prescribed not to mention good medical advice to prevent such episodes.

## Management of Sex Partners:

Patient's past and current sex partners should be identified, evaluated, and treated.

Patient and partners are also instructed to abstain from sexual intercourse until complete cure is accomplished and symptoms resolved for all concerned. On rare occasions men may experience treatment failure due to resistance to metronidazole. Tinidazole is prescribed for favorable outcome.

# PART V
## Sexually Transmitted Diseases by Parasites and Ectoparasites

### 1. Lice Infestation- Pediculosis
### A. Pubic Lice
### Pediculosis pubis - Phthirus pubis

Pediculosis pubis, a common infestation of adults is transmitted by sexual and physical intimacy. Pubic louse, an obligate parasite usually targets pubic/genital area but can also spread to chest hair, eyebrows, and eyelashes. Lice infestation may cause un-easiness, itching, and a creepy feeling. The tiny lice barely visible to the naked eye are popularly known as crabs for their oblong shape that resembles crab. Nonsexual transmission among children and adults can happen. Poor hygiene and physical contact among people living in crowded environments such as slums, institutional living, and homeless shelters increase risk for transmission. Lice infestation is much more common in tropics and subtropics than temperate weather zones.

## Figure 7
### Pediculosis pubis – Phthirus pubis

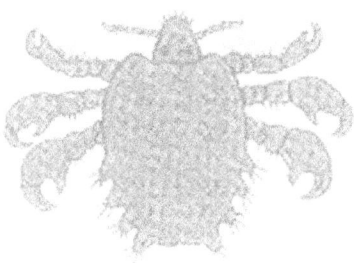

Pubic Louse

## Transmission:

- Infested persons can readily transmit pubic lice to their sex partners.
- Persons infested with pubic lice can transmit tiny parasites to their friends and family by physical contact.
- Sharing bedding, towels, and clothing can transmit lice.
- Sharing comb, hat, and other personal items increases risk.
- Children can acquire pediculosis by intimate physical contact with infected adults and play-mates.

## Symptoms:

Most people notice lice infestation in and around genital/ pubic and anal area within days after exposure. Lice rapidly multiply, lay hundreds of eggs which stick to the base of pubic hair, hair on the lower abdomen, and upper thighs. The silvery white eggs called nits adhere to pubic hair at the hair-skin junction. As nits hatch infestation may spread to rest of the body such as arm-pits, beard, chest, mustache, eyebrows, and scalp hair. Most people have symptoms as described below.

- Lice infestation may cause mild to severe itching of the anogenital area.
- Pubic lice cause tingling feeling around the penis, vagina, and anus.
- Noticeable tiny brown spots (louse excrement) resembling dried blood specs on the undergarment.
- Severe infestation may cause awkward creepy discomfort and restlessness.

## Diagnosis:

Most adults can feel and sense pubic lice infestation. Though such admission is never made in public, sex partners normally share such information and exchange remedies.

Most adults seek medical advice and treatment from health care providers.

Healthcare providers examine genital/anal area for nits and lice. Nits are gently scraped for visual examination under microscope to confirm the presence of pubic lice. The procedure is fast and painless.

## Treatment:

Persons who seek professional care are diagnosed as above and treated with topical creams or oral medications or both as listed below.

## Topical creams or lotions recommended for treatment:

- Malathion 0.5% cream or lotion.
- Permethrin 1% cream.
- Pyrethrins with piperonyl butoxide.

Usually creams or lotions are directly applied to the affected areas and washed off after 10-15 minutes.

## Oral Medication:

Ivermectin 250 ug, repeated in 2 weeks.

Over the counter remedies are also available in the U.S. If using such remedies, carefully read labels before application. If it is an oral dose follow instructions and take recommended dose only. If eye brows/eye lashes require lotion/cream application, be extremely careful. Apply occlusive ophthalmic ointments only as prescribed by your eye doctor. Skin lotion/creams may be harmful to your eyes.

Pregnant women and breastfeeding mothers are treated with above listed creams or lotions only. Ivermectin oral or topical regimen is not recommended for pregnant and breastfeeding women. On rare occasions if patients don't respond to common medications, Lindane (lotion or shampoo) may be prescribed. Lindane has some very serious side effects for adults, children, and infants therefore extreme precautions are necessary. Lindane must be applied "just as prescribed" by the physician.

## Remedies and Prevention:

- Bedding, clothing, garments, and used towels from infected persons must be separated, washed with detergent, hot water, and put through hot dry cycle.
- Avoid sex and physical contact with infected persons.
- Avoid hugging, kissing, and other forms of intimate playful acts.
- Infected persons must avoid sexual and physical intimacy with friends and family.
- Sex partner selection and personal hygiene can also help.
- Fumigation of living areas is not recommended.

## Follow – Up:
Patients are usually evaluated 8- 15 days after initial treatment or sooner if necessary. If lice and nits are still present treatment must be extended or an alternate cream or lotion recommended for favorable outcome. Usually treatment failure is attributed to misdiagnosis, failure to follow medical advice, reinfection, and rarely drug resistance.

## Management of Sex Partners:
Sex partners who had contact with patients are identified, evaluated, and treated as above. Total abstinence is recommended from all involved while receiving treatment until symptoms fully resolve. Follow-up visits and retreatment if

necessary are also offered. Lice infestation is easy to detect, inexpensive to treat, and most important of all causes no permanent damage or disability.

Patients with pediculosis pubis are usually evaluated for other STDs as a precaution. Most sexually active people with multiple partners are at greater risk for common STDs such as HIV, herpes, syphilis, and others.

## B. Body Lice
## Pediculus humanus corpus

Body lice usually found among people with poor body hygiene and those living in crowded institutions and close housing environments such as communal living, nursing home, retirement community, orphanage, penitentiary, dormitory, slums, and homeless shelters. Body lice can cause infections such as relapsing fever, trench fever, and typhus. Infestation is not sexually transmitted - physical proximity not sexual intimacy will do you in.

### Figure 8
### Pediculus humanus corpus

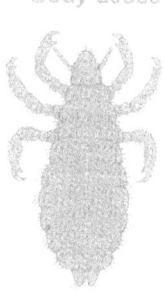
Body Louse

## C. Head Lice
## Pediculus humanus capitis

Head lice infestation is a common scourge for school age children. Head lice infestation is spread by personal contact among children and rarely among adults. Children sharing combs, brushes, hats, and personal items are at greater risk of acquiring head lice infestation. If not resolved promptly lice may infest eyebrows, eyelashes, and facial hair among boys. Head lice infestation is not sexually transmitted.

### Figure 9
### Pediculus humanus capitis

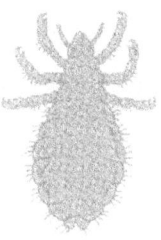

Head Louse

## 2. Scabies
### Skin Infection
### Scabies Itch Mite - Sarcoptes scabiei

Scabies, a highly contagious mite infestation is caused by a skin parasite Sarcoptes scabiei. Infestation usually results in pruritus all over the body. Newly infected person may take weeks to develop tiny pus filled reddish pimples (pruritus) on the skin that brings on intense itching. But for subsequent infection pruritus and itching is swift – usually within 24 hours. Patients' swift pruritic response and other clinical symptoms result from hypersensitivity to the itch mite, its feces, and eggs.

The female mite burrows under the skin, deposits hundreds of eggs which hatch within days. The baby mites or larvae continue to spread infestation.

Scabies skin infection is common among adults and children. Adults frequently acquire scabies by sexual contact but children usually by non-sexual means. Scabies is prevalent in tropics and sub tropics than in temperate weather zones. More than 300 million people worldwide come down with scabies each year.

## Transmission:

Transmission of itch mite can happen by physical contact as described below:

- Infected adults can transmit scabies to sex partners and their physical contacts.
- Most children, household members, nursing home residents, prison inmates, people living in crowded and institutionalized environment are at higher risk to acquire scabies by physical contact with an infected person.
- People sharing clothing, bedding, towels, and personal items can acquire scabies.

- Casual contact in the work place, place of worship, and social gathering are less likely to cause scabies infestation but it's wise to avoid physical contact with infected people.

## Prevention of Transmission:

- Avoid sex and physical contact with infected people.
- Avoid hugging, holding hands, shaking hands, and physical contact with infected people.
- Avoid sharing clothes, bedding, towels, razor, comb, brush, hat, and other personal items with infected people.
- Infected people must avoid physical contact with friends and neighbors.
- Parents must protect children from infected people.
- Parents/guardians of infected children should seek medical help ASAP and prevent transmission to others by isolating children from playmates until resolution of infestation.

## Symptoms:

Scabies patients usually develop pruritus, the characteristic symptom. However sensitization is a pre-requisite for pruritus. Sensitization process among people who get infected for the very first time may take weeks. But for subsequent reinfection pruritus may be swift – usually within 24 hours.

Symptoms listed below may appear within 2 -4 weeks upon exposure to itch mite.

- Initial immune response is intense itching followed by appearance of tiny reddish pus filled rashes.
- Itching is most intense in the webs between fingers, wrist, elbow, armpits, beltline, upper and lower part of the buttocks.
- Genital (penis and scrotum) itching in men is intense, painful, and embarrassing.
- In women, itching is severe in the vulva, buttocks, around the nipples, and breasts.
- Heavy infestation of scabies may affect every part of the body including scalp.
- Itching and urge to itch becomes compulsive soon after shower and much worse at night.

Children may not develop characteristic symptoms. Unlike adults, small children initially produce fluid filled blisters or red rashes on the face. Children often scratch skin rashes and develop bacterial infection. People taking medication containing steroids may have symptoms suppressed but symptoms eventually appear.

## Diagnosis:

Classic burrowing tunnels of itch mite and patient's urge to itch are significant diagnostic indicators to determine scabies infestation. Doctors may also examine skin scraping under the microscope. Presence of itch mite and eggs confirm scabies. Patients receiving therapy containing steroids for any condition usually don't itch nor have the urge to itch therefore difficult to diagnose other than microscopic examination of skin scrapings.

## Treatment:

Scabies is treated with topical creams and lotions such as:

**Permethrin (5%) Cream:** Applied to all parts of the body from neck down and washed off 8-12 hours after application. **Lindane (1%) Lotion:** Applied and washed off as above. Lindane is not routinely prescribed to patients because of serious side effects. It is occasionally prescribed to patients who are allergic to other medications.

## Oral regimen:

**Ivermectin (200ug/kg):** Initial treatment resolves scabies for most patients. However patients must be reevaluated by a follow up visit in two weeks to confirm treatment success.

Pregnant and breastfeeding women should not be prescribed lindane and ivermectin because of adverse effects to the unborn and the newborn.

Lindane and ivermectin are toxic therefore not recommended for infants and young children.

In addition to the above patients may be prescribed antihistamines for itch prevention. Patients may continue episodal itch for up to 2- 3 weeks even after scabies resolution.

## Remedial and Preventive Measures:

- Family members, sex partners, and friends should be examined and treated promptly as preventive and control measures.
- Bedding, clothing, and other garments should be washed with hot water and hot dry cycle.
- If washing clothes as described above is not possible such clothes should be kept away from

patients' body contact for at least 72 hours. Fumigation of clothes is not recommended.

- Itch mite has a short life span outside human skin therefore easy to exterminate.
- Clipping/cleaning fingernails of all infected/ treated people, especially children in any setting is helpful to prevent re-infestation and bacterial infection.

## Follow – UP:

Scabies is highly contagious that requires follow-up care and treatment. Some people may be contagious for 2 - 4 weeks even after treatment completion. To some treatment may not have been effective, wrongly applied, or simply failed. Follow – up evaluation and treatment with an alternate regimen is recommended for all such patients.

HIV positive and immune impaired people are at increased risk for severe form of infection known as crusted scabies or Norwegian scabies. Crusted scabies is hot bed for bacterial, viral, and other infections that should be aggressively treated in consultation with an infectious disease specialist.

HIV/AIDS and immune impaired patients are at much greater risk for treatment failure for variety of reasons therefore treated simultaneously with topical and oral regimens much longer or until completely free of symptoms.

## Management of Sex Partners:

Sexual, household, and personal contacts of patients in the preceding 30 days of diagnosis should be identified, evaluated, and treated if indicated. Household members, friends, and sex partners should be instructed to avoid contact with patients until everyone is treated and symptoms fully resolved.

## Scabies Outbreaks in Communities, Group Homes, Nursing Homes, and Residential Facilities:

Nursing homes, residential, and institutionalized settings are prone to scabies epidemic. Prevention and control of such an outbreak can be a monumental task. An effective strategy for such incidents must be developed. Coordination of resources, professional guidance by experts in the field, and community participation is absolutely essential to overcome such an epidemic. Residential population at risk should be counseled to avoid exposure.

In the event of an outbreak everyone may have to be provided presumptive treatment - oral/topical medications supported by diligent follow – up treatment and care until everyone is totally free of symptoms.

# PART VI
## Violence against Women and Children
## Sexuality – Male and Female
## Sex Offenses against Adults and Children
## Rape and Gang Rape
## Sexual Harassment
## Prevention of Crime and Repeat Offense
## Child Abuse – Physical and Sexual Abuse

## Sexuality – Male and Female

Sexuality is being identified inwardly and outwardly as male or female. We are born as male or female with rare exception of indeterminate sex. Characteristic physical differences obviously dictate our sexuality.

- Sexuality is what makes a person male or female.
- Sexuality is our "inner sense" and conviction.
- Sexuality is how one consciously and naturally behaves.

## Sexuality is defined and influenced by factors such as:

- Biological characteristics/factors and physical features influence and define sexuality.
- Cultural roles also define sexuality. Different cultures of the world dictate and promote unique public behavior, attitude expected of males and females. Such customs may vary from culture to culture.
- Psychological factors involve personal/family based beliefs, emotions, and expression of

feelings in private or public. Much has to do with how we perceive the way society treats/ responds to such form of sexuality. Most societies and cultures have unique ways of expressing sexuality.

Persons' sex or gender differences influence the gender role that person usually assumes and publicly displays. Gender based behavior is naturally expected in society, school, work place, and wide range of other places and situations.

Most pre-pubertal boys and girls anxious to grow up to be adolescents develop own personal beliefs, sociocultural roles, likes, dislikes, and display unique personal identity. Boys and girls of pubertal age also feel and display intense emotional and physical attraction towards persons of opposite sex. Parents, religion, media, and society at large emphasize and influence gender related outlook, attitude, and acceptable social/sexual behavior. Awareness of gender roles such as masculine behavior in boys and feminine characteristics in girls are naturally accepted and practiced. Society at large rewards culturally acceptable behavior and mercilessly penalizes misbehavior.

Children grow out of puberty, a process that involves so much to so many but ultimate result is predictable self-expression of sexuality. Some may follow traditional values yet some may defy tradition completely. Each person by design and instinct develops special interests, fantasies, preferences, unique desires/needs, and distinctive sexual values. Most youngsters also look to develop relationship with persons of opposite sex out of strong feelings of love that may lead to permanent relationship and marriage. Persons who are sexually attracted to one another are in love – an intertwined intimate relationship.

Forms of sexual expression such as emotional bonding and love may vary widely among countries and cultures. However public expression may be limited to:

- Holding hands.
- Hugging and kissing.
- Social outing such as picnics, indoor or outdoor parties.
- Attend sports events, games, musicals, movies, and theatre.

Other forms of sexual expression include intimate relationship such as:

- Living together in a committed relationship.
- Getting married – a legal arrangement.
- Raising family according to existing cultural norms.

Most countries, cultures, and societies follow self – imposed traditions and customs. In some countries such as India where arranged marriage is prevalent parents choose spouse for their children. Western cultures such as Europe and U.S. usually leave such decision to prospective couple.

Current trend in most countries and cultures is that each person may decide how and when to express desire for love, intimacy, and companionship – all part of sexual expression. Most people are influenced in their decision by learned/accepted values from family, friends, peers, and not the least of all - religion.

Love, sex, and relationship between two consenting adults is too complex to deal with and not the subject for this guide. However this guide in part is about the dark, violent side of sex and sexual behavior/relationship such as sexual assault, and abuse. Unpleasant consequences of poor choice, sex and sexual conduct that may cause pain, suffering, victimization, and STDs is the real focus.

## Sex Offenses against Adults and Children
## Rape and Gang Rape

Sexual violence is a serious offense yet is common in every culture, most countries, and communities. Almost all countries have laws that impose heavy monetary penalties and severe punishment to perpetrators. Yet tragically sexual assaults such as rape and sodomy are on the rise in all parts of the world. My beloved country of birth, India is in the midst of a tsunami of horrific sexual crimes not to mention several recent barbaric gang rapes which received world – wide condemnation.

Scheming perpetrators execute sexual assault(s) by clever planning and timing at a pre-designated place in order to "protect" self. Some most common sexual assaults are listed below.

### Rape:
Rape is sexual assault, an act of violence, and domination committed against that person's will. Rape is humiliating and brutalizing a victim that may involve anal, oral, and vagi-

nal penetration. Some rapists physically abuse, torture, and even kill their victims. Men, women and children may be victimized but most victims are women, minor underage girls, and children.

Victims of rape do not anticipate crime until it happens. Most victims are familiar or know their attacker(s). Such unwanted/unsolicited forced sexual assaults can be described as:

1. **Date rape:** Forced intercourse/penetration with another person while on social event such as social outing, date, and courtship.
2. **Marital rape:** Forced intercourse with the unwilling spouse.
3. **Statutory rape:** Refers to sexual intercourse with an underage person. In most States in the U.S. statutory rape is a felony of the first degree.

## Gang Rape:

Approximately 10-15% of estimated sexual assaults are gang-rapes. Gang-rape, also known as group or party rape is committed by multiple men against helpless women, usually under the influence of alcohol and drugs. Compromised state of mind can contribute to such an unusual barbaric crime. Most gang rapes are pre-meditated and a few because of "opportunity knocking". College campuses and poor urban neighborhoods frequently report such crimes. Yet most rapes and gang rapes occur near surroundings or places victim(s) frequently shop, play, and visit. Gang rape may be committed for just pleasure, revenge, or simply nothing better to do!

Rape can be a double edged sword for rapist(s) and victim(s). Underlying infection can be transmitted aggravating the same for everyone involved. If one is infected with an STD of any origin, others will most likely acquire that infection. Many innocent men, women, and children suffer this heart wrenching misfortune and many more continue to struggle with disease such as herpes, HIV/AIDS, and syphilis just to name a few.

For legal purposes other sex offenses against women and children can be described as follows:

## Sexual battery:

Sexual battery is defined as an act whereby the offender by virtue of his/her position, relationship, or status knowingly entices/coerces the other person to submit by any means that would prevent resistance to the act of sexual abuse. Most victims of sexual battery feel trapped, find it impossible to escape, and even choose not to report the crime out of fear of unknown. Victims fear humiliation, pain, physical abuse, torture, disease, blackmail, and even death. Anyone can be forced to such a scheme. In many states in the U.S., sexual battery is a felony of the third degree. If the victim is under 16 years of age (minor) the offense is a felony of the fourth degree. The seriousness of crime with minor is also judged by perpetrator's age.

## Gross sexual imposition:

Gross sexual imposition is a pre-meditated crime. The predator tricks the other person to submit by force or threat of force. The scheming offender may also force the victim or influence victim's judgment by administering alcohol, drugs, or any other substance to achieve desired goals. In a crime of this kind the offender may exploit victim's age, physical or mental condition, or any other disability that suits best. The reluctant victim is then repeatedly subjected to the whims of the offender.

## Importuning:

Importuning is a crime committed by an adult soliciting sex from a minor. In the U.S., it is a crime to engage in any form of sexual activity with a person who is under 13 years of age.

## Voyeurism:

An act that is secretly or surreptitiously trespass/invade privacy of a person(s) by eavesdropping or spying for sexual arousal and gratification. The offender may fulfill deviant desires by videotape, film, pictures, or recording conversations under compromised situations.

## Public indecency:

A person is considered an offender for reckless conduct and behavior involving acts of indecency in physical proximity to people who are not immediate members of his/her family.

- Offender exposing private body parts to lure girls/women/boys/men.
- Engage in untoward sexual activity or masturbation.
- Engage in unseemly inappropriate sexual activity or misconduct that an ordinary observer may deem it to be inappropriate.

Most sex offenses may involve forced sexual acts/ behaviors and penetration. Clearly sexual assault is an act of aggression that violates privacy, and moral/social sensitivities of victims.

## Sexual Harassment

Sexual harassment consists of unwelcome/unsolicited sexual advances, inappropriate requests for sexual favors, and subtle physical and verbal overtures. Gender biased blatant hurtful behavior is also considered to be yet another form of sexual harassment. Women are far more likely to be victims though rarely men may find to be at the receiving end. Sexual harassment can happen in any setting – social, work place environment, or any other. Employment related sexual harassment may include:

1. Quid pro quo can occur when person(s) in authority requests/demands sexual favors from an employee in exchange for getting hired, not getting fired, job advantage such as flexible hours, promotion, and better working conditions.
2. Hostile environment may include explicit environment of sexuality, obscene behavior, and presence of pornographic material suggestive of obvious intent.

Most developed and developing countries have laws to protect people (mostly women) from sexual harassment in the work place. In the U.S., the Civil Rights Act of 1964 recognizes sexual harassment as a form of sexual discrimination and holds employers responsible to uphold the law. Therefore all U. S. employers diligently develop an effective policy to deal with sexual harassment complaints and educate employees accordingly rather than face legal and monetary penalties. Most states in the U.S. also have laws designed to deter and prevent sexual crimes against women and children. Purpose for such laws is clearly to accomplish:

- Encourage victims to report sexual abuse, harassment, and rape.
- Promote truth-finding process and exclude inappropriate evidence.
- Victims' sexual privacy and protection from undue harassment.
- Discourage rape victims being tried and prosecuted.
- Perpetrators caught and punished under existing state/federal laws.

Most jurisdictions in the U.S. treat sexual crimes against women and children with great sensitivity. Victims are treated with compassion and concern for safety. Local police have experience and training to respond to such crimes in a professional manner. Accurate documentation from get go is essential along with other emergency services such as bringing the victim(s) to hospital/clinic ASAP, first aid if necessary, and collection of appropriate forensic evidence.

Upon victim's arrival to any medical facility experienced professionals deal with medical emergency as described under "Initial Evaluation for Sexual Assault Victims" in this chapter.

The judiciary hand in glove with police, sheriff's department, and social welfare agencies expedite trial and coordinate all available assistance to victims of crime. Speedy resolution is a deterrent to such crimes.

### Prevention of Crime and Repeat Offence

Most communities in the U.S. provide education and counseling to citizens especially women and children concerning rape, sexual assault, and other sex crimes. Such knowledge also brings awareness and a watchful eye to foresee impending tragedy. On occasion when a predator is loose or seen in the community police warn the citizens to be aware and watchful as a precaution.

U.S. also maintains offender registry that can alert communities nationwide. When criminals move out or move into a community residents are notified. Critical information and changes are promptly upgraded and also made available to concerned citizens via internet and mail:

- Sex offender's gender, age, name, recent/old picture, and previous/current address.
- Type of sex offense committed such as Tier 3 (Serious crime), Tier 2 (less serious crime) and Tier 1 (even lesser serious crime).
- Tier 3 criminal is required to register with local police every 90 days for life. Change of residence must be periodically updated for life.
- Tier 2 criminal is required to register with local police twice a year. Change of residence updated at regular intervals.

- Tier 1 criminal is required to register with local police once a year. Change of residence updated as per local law.

When new sex offender(s) arrives in any community, local authorities promptly notify neighbors via internet and mail so all may take precautions, protect self/family, and avoid unpleasant consequences.

Local, state, and federal government has an obligation and responsibility to control and conquer the menace of sex crimes. Strong laws in the books and stiff penalties alone are not enough. Experts advocate sex education for children and teens as one such important step. A well thought out program can be an attractive option. Two such programs listed below are proposed by opposing ideologues. Though programs have major differences common ground can be found for the greater good of our children. Protecting innocent children and women from physical violence and sex abuse should be a priority for all.

Teachers can encourage open and honest discussion of sexuality, acceptable sexual behavior, and promote greater awareness of do's and don'ts among children at an early age. Communities in the U.S. are free to introduce any program that suits best. Most school districts are well-equipped to develop and teach the youngsters as per community guidelines.

## 1. Abstinence only program:

Righteous moral approach explored. Disregard to some critical issues such as listed below makes this program less attractive.

- Greater emphasis on abstinence until marriage
- Disregard for barrier methods to avoid pregnancy, STIs, and HIV.
- Less emphasis on education, communication, and health benefits of safe sex.
- Greater role for parents with issues such as communication, counseling, and sex education.

Some parents are not familiar with current advances, innovations, and age appropriate communication skills. Some parents are reluctant to talk to their children about sex for fear of promoting promiscuity.

## 2. Comprehensive program:

This program proposes detailed approach to all issues involving sexuality and sex. The program can be introduced to children at a very young age. Community leaders are free to introduce the program with changes to adhere to community values.

Explicit goal of each program is to protect innocent children from predators, human traffickers, and sex offenders. Children need to be aware of constant dangers therefore must be trained to look out. Teachers can best prepare them as described below.

- Children learn that sex is what makes males and females different. The obvious distinction clearly defines proper sex-roles.
- Respect for sexual identity is learned at a very young age.

- Youngsters learn healthy sexual behavior based on community values, acceptable social practices with emphasis on respect for privacy and human dignity.
- Proper behavior to protect privacy, self-esteem, and a "wholesome" attitude taught early in life usually makes lasting impression.
- Function of each organ of human body including sex organs is explained.
- Medically accurate information taught to children at age appropriate level can greatly benefit.
- Children should be taught that babies come from their parents but not confused with details.
- Older children, ages 8 – 11 are prepared for puberty such as anticipated changes in male and female bodies.
- Questions about sex and related issues explained as science.
- Moral, ethical issues along with respect for opposite sex are explained based on community values.
- Students beyond puberty are informed about individual responsibility related to sex, sexuality, dating, intimate relationship, and abstinence.
- High school juniors and seniors understand topics such as birth control, appropriate sexual behavior, commitment, and marriage.

- Consequences of reckless irresponsible behavior are core subject for sex education.
- Consequences of unwanted, unsolicited, repulsive sexual advances/behavior emphacised.
- Consequences of sexual assault, sex offense, and other devious acts can hurt victims and perpetrators.
- Respect for law of the land and respect for opposite sex is a learned behavior – children usually pay much attention to their teacher(s) and follow advice.

Some experts also suggest that sex education be initiated in kindergarten and continued through high school and beyond. Curriculum can be developed so children become familiar with many aspects of sexuality at a gradual pace.

Students usually trust teachers and overcome myths. Sex education can be devised so children can understand and accept community standards fully. The program, if taught by experienced educators can make lasting impact. Age appropriate subject matter must be carefully selected and tastefully presented to students for maximum benefit. These programs can be taught to students of all ages with parental consent and active participation.

Sexual reproduction is a process of recreation among higher animals and humans. For humans sex is much more than just reproduction. The choice to have children involves unshakable commitment, love, strong bonding, and permanent social impact. Love for person(s) of opposite sex, deep desire for sex results in marriage and lasting covenant.

In most modern western societies boys and girls grow up together, become familiar with one another, bond, and develop love, respect, and intimate relationship with a person of their choice. Steady courting can promote commitment and much love. Emotional and sexual attraction ultimately can result in marriage.

Physical, psychological, medical, long term and short term discomfort, pain, and suffering for victims of abuse is a serious issue. Some victims may learn to overcome but most require much care and counseling – usually for life.

For victims of sexual abuse life and living must continue without fear, feeling of guilt, shame, and social stigma. For most victims of sexual assault such horrors may bring on emotional and psychological distress. Pain, suffering, depression, and physical scarring for life are also common.

Most sexual assaults are not reported to the police because such crimes are committed by persons known to the victims. Rarely strangers take advantage of innocent children and women however with education/training some such crimes can be prevented.

Most child victims are likely to confide in their teachers and intimate friends in part due to perceived parental fear. Some victims may not even talk about the incident out of fear that perpetrator may strike again. Delay in seeking legal/medical help may work in perpetrator's favor and crimes may go unpunished. Most traumatized victims also face the scourge of common STDs such as chlamydia, gonorrhea, herpes, hepatitis, syphilis, and life threatening HIV. In some cases help may come little too late.

Children who learn normal sexual behavior may instinctively report abnormal deviant sexual overtures to parents, siblings, teachers, and police. This important initial step may open doors for medical help, prevention/management of STDs, blood borne viral infections, and critical emergency needs such as resolving conception.

## Initial Evaluation for Sexual Assault Victims

Survivors of sexual assault need prompt compassionate medical and psychological care. In the U.S. experienced professionals evaluate urgent individual needs and provide support in an effort to minimize further physical and mental trauma caused by sexual assault not only to victims but to victim's families as well.

In the U. S. all 50 states and protective territories have clear legal guidelines and clinical procedures to protect and support victims, victim's dignity, and privacy. Laws in all states strictly limit evidentiary use of survivor's previous sexual history. Previously acquired STDs as part of an anticipated effort to undermine survivor's credibility are also protected by law. Evidentiary privilege against disclosure of any part of the examination or treatment is also strictly enforced in all states. Testing for STDs may be deferred even though appropriate specimens are collected and maintained under strict legal custody.

Some common infections such as BV, chlamydia, gonorrhea, trichomoniasis, and yeast are most frequently identified among women. These are prevalent conditions not necessarily acquired as a result of rape. STDs such as herpes, hepatitis (B & C), HIV, syphilis, and a few others are a serious cause of concern for all victims of sexual assault. A thorough post assault examination is an important initial step and opportunity to identify (if any), treat, and prevent such STDs. Therefore victim must be rushed to the nearest medical center/clinic as delay may hamper examination and treatment. It's an inconvenient and emergency situation but healthcare professionals in the U.S. have experience dealing with traumatic situations of this kind. Always expect compassionate, understanding, and supportive healthcare professionals on your side. Careful thorough evaluation, physical examination, psychological assessment, and counseling are provided along with expert professional medical treatment.

## Initial evaluation requires the Following:

**Brief History:** Name, address, date of birth, and any other relevant information such as parents/guardians or responsible party.

**Reason for visit:** Emergency-information such as bruises, bleeding, pain, swelling, itching, discharge, malodor etc.

Males and females can have different symptoms at different sites – provide full graphic details.

**Type of Sexual Assault:** Perpetrator's sex (male or female), nature of assault such as abuse, molesting, rape and any other. If multiple persons involved clearly state how many. Examiner(s) may have specific questions concerning the incident – answer as best as you can.

**Sexual History:** This may be difficult but be truthful – information will be strictly confidential and used only to develop a treatment plan best for you.

**Past/current STDs:** Be truthful. Past or current HIV, HSV, HPV, syphilis, and any other disease will help treat you appropriately.

**Immunization (s) for any STDs:** HPV, Hepatitis A & B, and any other.

**Drugs and Medications:** State if illicit drugs and alcohol are involved. Information concerning victims' drug allergies, antibiotic resistance, and current antiviral medications are critical to treat and manage current incident/accident.

Victim or victims' parent or guardians may have to communicate with medical staff so initial evaluation is complete and victim is ready for initial examination. If victim is a minor parent/guardian will be asked to be present during examination and beyond. Initial examination may be extensive and time consuming. Based on history and reason for visit variety of procedures and blood tests may be performed for definitive diagnosis.

**Males:** Provide details, describe as best as you can so examiner, doctor/nurse clearly understand all that has happened. Location of pain, organ(s) affected.

**Females:** Provide Gynecological history (as asked). Pregnancy, menstruation, oral contraceptives, supplements, surgical procedures, and other critical information.

## Initial Examination

Medical facilities in the U.S. have protocol and procedures in place for all medical emergency situations including sexual assault. In instances of sexual assault the examination may include (but not limited to) the following:

## Female Victims:

- Wet mount can detect BV, yeast, and trichomoniasis.
- Gram Stain for N. gonorrhoeae.

- Vaginal swab (s) for gonorrhea, chlamydia, and other suspect pathogens.
- Recommended specimen for NAATs for chlamydia and gonorrhea.

Multiple specimens must be secured from all sites of penetration or attempted sites of penetration such as anus, mouth, and vagina.

Multiple vials (tubes) of blood samples must be secured for testing STDs such as hepatitis (A, B, C), HIV, herpes, and syphilis.

## Male victims (men and boys):

Men and young boys are also frequent victims of sexual assault. Examination of male victims can be exhaustive. Following specimens may be secured for diagnosis and treatment.

- Wet prep from anorectal area for yeast and bacteria.
- Anorectal swabs for gram stain to detect gonorrhea.
- Specimen for NAATs from all sites of penetration or attempted penetration.
- Blood samples for testing STDs such as hepatitis (A, B, C), HIV, herpes, and syphilis.

Initial evaluation of males and females must include accurate documentation of all findings, collection of all relevant specimens for forensic examination, management of potential pregnancy among females, and psychological/ physical trauma.

## Follow-Up Examination for Victims

Follow-up examination is critically important in all cases of sexual abuse. Victims need extensive general and specialized individual care and counseling. Post assault examination is recommended 2-4 weeks after the initial examination. This provides an opportunity for health-care givers to reexamine victims, share information, and determine future course for treatment plan as listed below.

- Determine progress if any, diagnose new infections, comfort/counsel victim(s) and immediate family.
- Better assessment of risk factors for serious infections such as HIV, hepatitis (B&C), herpes, and syphilis can be made based on available data and response to initial treatment.
- Complete hepatitis B vaccination if initial regimen was administered during previous/initial visit.
- Assess adverse effects and compliance of prescribed treatment.
- Most women of child bearing age and young girls face the traumatic issue of pregnancy. Adequate counseling, treatment, and care must be provided during follow-up visit (s). Pregnancy resolution can be a moral/ethical issue.
- In most sexual assault incidents prophylactic antibiotics and medications are provided to victims for anticipated infections such as chlamydia, gonorrhea, hepatitis, herpes, HIV, syphilis, and others during initial examination. Follow-up examination is useful to determine

progress and treatment changes if indicated. Treatment may be continued for some and discontinued for others.

- Victim's follow-up visit is also an occasion for clinicians and medical staff to initiate helpful dialogue concerning other STDs. Initial symptoms for such STDs must be clearly explained so the victims may seek help and prompt care.

In the event healthcare givers and medical staff conclude outside counseling services are necessary proper arrangements should be made as per guidelines. Future visits scheduled as medically necessary.

In all instances of sexual assault much attention must be paid to assailants' health status to cope with potential physical and psychological impact to the victim(s). Survivors must be professionally counseled and adequately prepared for imminent risk factors for serious infections such as HIV, herpes, chlamydia, syphilis, and others. Survivors' fears and concerns must be carefully considered and best available options recommended. Assailant's medical history and mental health must be documented in order to support/counsel victim(s) appropriately.

- Evaluate and document all issues related to assault such as assailant's physical and mental health.
- Assailant must be tested for STDs such as HIV, hepatitis (A, B, & C), herpes, chlamydia, gonorrhea, syphilis, and others if indicated.
- Based on thorough physical examination determine risk for HIV, herpes, syphilis and other STDs to the

victim. If need be, specialists must be brought in for more extensive informative consultation.

- Survivors may require medical advice and peace of mind concerning HIV and herpes threat: properly guide and relieve concerns/ fears by proposing benefits of antiviral prophylactic therapy. Side effects of such medications also need to be explained.
- Victims in most cases agree for aggressive prophylactic management but may not fully comply. Therefore they must be provided with adequate supply of such medications and warned of dangers of non-compliance.
- Immediate and lasting effects of medications vary among individuals therefore all persons taking prophylactic antiviral medications need to be monitored closely. Physical examination and blood tests should be performed at intervals, HIV antibody test done at 6 weeks, 3 months, and 6 months post assault.
- If the assailant is positive for hepatitis B victim is promptly administered vaccine or HGB (or both) ASAP.
- More follow-up visits must be scheduled for counseling, consultation, and management if indicated.

Victims' progress and eventual normalcy is always a priority for caring professionals. Victims and immediate family therefore should take medical advice seriously for favorable outcome.

# Child Abuse
## Physical and Sexual Abuse

Mistreatment of a child by an adult such as parent, caregiver(s), neighbor(s), and even stranger(s) is a simple definition of child abuse. Child abuse can be inflicted in many forms such as denial of food, shelter (basic needs), emotional/psychological/ mental trauma, physical, and sexual exploitation. Child abuse is widespread in every part of the world. No country, developed or poor is completely free of such scourge to the future generation. Mistreatment of a child by an adult, caregiver, or parents in the guise of correcting bad behavior by inhumane means is also a form of child abuse. Child trafficking, another form of abuse is a crime yet it's prevalent in many countries. In India more than 45,000 children go missing each year. An accurate number of abducted and missing children worldwide are not available but presumed to be astronomical.

Thousands of innocent children are abducted, abused, exploited, brutalized, raped, forced to live under inhumane conditions, and even killed year after year. Sweet dreams and bold aspirations denied for these tender hearts forever: all for selfish instant gratification.

Cultural and social compulsions coupled with presumed economic security is yet another reason many families in China, India and few other countries opt for baby boys. Baby girls are abandoned, discarded, abused, mutilated, and even killed. Many parents abort baby girls as soon as they are able to determine baby's sex. Laws exist to deter such crude, inhumane procedure in several Indian states but authorities and clinics conveniently look the other way for a petty bribe rather than search their conscience to deliver justice. Most common forms of child abuse are listed below.

- Child neglect: denial of basic needs such as food, clothing, and shelter.
- Infliction of emotional, psychological pain and suffering.
- Life threatening physical violence such as severe beating, burning with hot rods, cigarette butts, and mutilation.
- Acts such as throwing children with intent to harm, lock/force children in closets, inhabitable environments, and rooms with no light or ventilation.
- Pour boiling water or force – drowning, strangulation, and choking.
- Suffocate under heat or objects such as pillows, bedding, and blankets.
- Gross sexual abuse including molesting and penetration.
- Forced child labor yet another form of child abuse is a serious social problem in many countries especially in India.

People engaged in child abuse find unique ways to "discipline and punish" children for behaviors they deem inappropriate.

Sexual abuse and exploitation of children is discussed in this guide as that involves serious life threatening STDs. Identification of such infections among children is critically important. Experienced healthcare givers can detect sexual abuse by the following symptoms in a child.

- Identification of any sexually transmitted disease(s) in children beyond neonatal phase is suggestive of sexual abuse.
- Postnatal gonorrhea, herpes, HIV, and syphilis are due to sexual abuse.
- Presence of genital warts alone does not confirm (only suspect) sexual abuse. Some non - abused children may have genital warts which may eventually disappear.
- Genital or rectal infection among children born to mothers with genital chlamydial infection may not be due to sexual abuse. Thorough physical examination can rule out abuse.
- Some abused children may acquire bacterial vaginosis. Presence of BV alone does not indicate abuse. Appropriate tests may determine the source of BV.
- Children may acquire hepatitis B from caregivers who are carriers of HBV and not by sexual abuse alone.
- Trichomonas may be identified among some children. Though it's less likely to be the result of sexual abuse, confirmation is necessary.

All states and protective territories in the U.S. have laws to protect children. Child abuse must be reported promptly to authorities by law. Childcare givers, healthcare providers, childcare experts/psychologists, social workers, and teachers must report any suspect abuse to state and local agency by law. In some states attorneys, coroners, ministers and priests are legally bound to report suspect child abuse. Neighbors, friends, and family reporting child abuse are protected by immunity from prosecution. Protecting nation's precious resource – our children is a priority for all. All communities, cities big and small have 24 hour hot-line to report crimes against children. Child abuse, endangerment, and neglect MUST BE REPORTED to the local/state agencies BY LAW.

United States is a leader in developing support programs for children of all forms of abuse as described above. The U.S. congress established The National Center on Child Abuse and Neglect in 1974. The center was reorganized in 1996 to support programs that deal with child abuse as the office on Child Abuse and Neglect, a division of The Children's Bureau, under the U.S. department of Health and Human Services (HHS). Episodes reported and identified as child abuse are promptly investigated and remedies suggested by state welfare experts. Protecting children from all forms of abuse, a noble cause that need to be vigorously pursued worldwide.

## Examination of Children and Pre-pubertal Girls

This process involves tremendous patience, skill, and expertise. Most children unaware of tragic serious situation at hand may adversely react out of anxiety and fear. Acute pain, discomfort, inconvenience, and presence of strangers can inflict even more of both. Therefore serious efforts must be made to protect the child in order to avoid yet another traumatic encounter. Only experienced medical personnel should visually inspect the child. It may be quite appropriate for parent/guardian to be present during such initial examination. A brief medical/personal history for boys and girls is obtained from parent/guardian prior initial examination as described already.

Initial evaluation involves collecting required oral, rectal, and vaginal specimens for analysis: procedure(s) may be time consuming and uncomfortable to the child and parent. Unique situation that forced the child to high risk must be pursued cautiously keeping in mind the social stigma and psychological trauma. Based on child's sex and initial visual inspection appropriate sites are selected for specimen collection (such as anorectal, oral, or vaginal). Sex appropriate specimens are collected for boys and girls. Pre-pubertal boys and girls require age appropriate specialized sample collection techniques.

Counseling by experienced professionals for abused children and parents throughout this ordeal is critically important. The parent/guardian is counseled in private and offered additional professional counseling if desired. Psychological evaluation should be provided with emphasis on individual child's mental and emotional needs. Childs recovery and family comfort must be the utmost priority in such situations.

## Initial Examination of the Child

- Visual inspection of anus, genitals, and mouth for bleeding, discharge, itching, lesions/ulcers, malodor, and warts is diligently performed and accurately documented.
- Evidence of oral, rectal, and vaginal penetration must be confirmed or ruled out:  appropriate specimens secured for laboratory testing.

- Symptoms or signs of STDs such as genital itching, pain, vaginal discharge, malodor, and urinary tract infection must be evaluated.
- Genital lesions/ulcers must be swabbed for bacterial, viral, and yeast identification.
- If vaginal penetration is confirmed blood and urine samples must be obtained from pubertal girls for pregnancy test.
- If symptoms for any STD exist, testing provisions must be made for all other STDs. This may require additional blood samples for antigen/antibody test and baseline titer(s).
- If child abuse occurred for an extended period diagnostic and treatment approach must be planned to provide maximum care with few visits to the clinic. Recent single episode of child abuse also requires good planning.
- It's critically important that assailant(s) is identified and tested for STDs, especially HIV, hepatitis group, herpes, syphilis, chlamydia, and gonorrhea.
- Infection of child's sibling or playmates for any STD should be an eye opener. This avenue is investigated in order to provide proper counseling and treatment.
- In the absence of definitive proof of child abuse/sexual assault parents or guardians may request tests for STDs. Test should be performed for their peace of mind and clear suspect behavior.

Above procedures must be performed prior to initiating treatment. Treatment may have to be delayed in some situations due to additional time required to obtain laboratory results. In all cases of child abuse only high specificity and reliable tests (regardless of cost) must be requested. Individualized professional care with most advanced diagnostic and treatment procedure(s) is critically important for child's recovery and well- being. All such procedures and treatment plans must be carefully scheduled for maximum benefit and convenience for the victim and family. Most victims and families affected by abuse are also in for a long frustrating legal battle not to mention psychological trauma and social stigma therefore all procedures performed and treatment plans developed should be well documented with such implications in mind.

## Follow-Up Examination for Children

Victimized children and their families require skilled professional support from get go. Most healthcare facilities and clinics in the U.S. have experienced personnel to provide such care. Follow-up care for children and their families is critically important: the process help prepare them to overcome anxeity, depression, and the fear of the unknown. Therefore parents/guardians must carefully follow social worker's and doctor's instructions during such visits. Parents/guardians may request special considerations based on child's unique situation. In order to feel free of social stigma, intimidation, and fear healthcare providers should welcome such request.

Follow-up visits must be scheduled based on individual child's special situation and unique requirements.

Counseling by professionals, clinicians, and auxiliary medical staff is an important part of treatment and care for the child. Much patience is required as clinic(s) performs routine and specialized procedures. In most cases child's parents/guardians may have to be professionally counseled and prepared for that rough road ahead. Follow-up visits may include repeat physical examination, several repeat procedures, blood, and urine tests. Healthcare providers may also perform following exploratory procedures.

- Anorectal examination for itching, bleeding, and lesions.
- Genital discharge (if any) collected for microscopic analysis and bacterial culture.
- Genital itching, bleeding, and malodor indicative of infection are followed up with additional tests.
- Genital ulcers/lesions and warts are swabbed for viral detection and culture.
- Mouth and throat lesions, sores, and malodor are checked for bacterial, viral, and yeast infections.
- Abused children must be monitored for hepatitis B, HIV, herpes, syphilis, or other infections.
- Assailant's health/disease status is reviewed to determine risk for victim(s). Even if slightest risk is evident presumptive treatment should be initiated and monitored with follow-up care.
- If hepatitis B is a concern but baseline (initial) tests are negative, such tests are repeated 6 weeks, 3, and 6 months after the initial tests.

- If HIV is a concern most caregivers may recommend post exposure presumptive treatment (PEP) with antiretroviral drugs. These drugs have serious side effects and the child may not tolerate the drug (s).
- HIV antibody blood test must be performed during the initial visit and at 6 weeks, 3, and 6 months.
- Caregivers also have an obligation to listen to parents/guardians concerns. Easing misgivings and fears may require additional procedures and tests for other common STDs. Child's future and protection from scarring requires critical assessment and careful consideration.

## HIV Post-exposure Assessment of Abused Children within 72 hours of Sexual Assault

Sexually abused children are at much greater risk for HIV. HIV antigen and antibody tests (baseline) are considered based on assailant's medical history or likelihood of HIV infection. Post exposure antiretroviral PEP within 72 hours is offered upon consultation with experts. Most children have minimal risk for serious adverse reactions therefore though presumed safety is sketchy perceived benefits may outweigh PEP treatment. Following suggestions must be considered when faced with a situation of such importance:

- Local epidemiology and assailant's risk for HIV.
- Assess child's risk post assault, consult specialists, and offer PEP only if indicated.

- Unproven efficacy and toxicity of antiretroviral PEP and potential benefits must be clearly explained to the parent/guardian.
- Age appropriate dosage and enough regimens until the next visit must be made available to the victim. Tolerance for medication is reevaluated and changes suggested as indicated.
- HIV antibody test is recommended at 0, 6 weeks, 3, and six months.

## Presumptive Treatment:

As already described sexually abused children may be at considerable risk for some common STDs. However if medical data suggest otherwise based on assailant's medical history presumptive post-exposure treatment may not be necessary. Incidence of STDs among children and pre-pubertal girls is relatively low therefore most caregivers may recommend regular follow-up visits as a precaution to ensure child's health. Such visits also provide an opportunity for parents/guardians to relate their concerns to health caregivers. Some parents/guardians may insist their child be treated in anticipation of certain disorders. Demand may be quite appropriate however caregiver may need additional time so a thorough review can be made to resolve the issue(s) based on all post assault diagnostic data on the child.

# PART VII
## STDs – Control and Prevention
## STD – Surveillance

Like the old saying "prevention is better than cure". Almost all sexually transmitted diseases can be prevented with rare exceptions. This Guide provides useful information for prevention and control of most common STDs. Living free of life threatening STDs can be rewarding. Safe sex brings much joy, immense pleasure, and a feeling of secure relationship among loving life-partners. Prevention of STDs saves lives, preserve good health, saves inconvenience, and financial drain.

Surest way to live free of STDs is abstinence altogether. You may also choose to limit your sexual prowess to one uninfected partner who in turn accommodates no one else but YOU.

Sexually active people can greatly reduce chances/risks for STDs by following effective protective measures as outlined in this section. Avoiding sexual contact with high risk individuals as already described will reduce risk. But there are several other ways to prevent STDs. Informed adults should strive to live healthy worry free sex life by adopting strategies best suited for their lifestyle. Factors such as demography, age groups at greater risk, alcohol and substance abuse contribute transmission of infection among sexually active people. The following multi-prong program can benefit all sexually active persons.

- Education combined with practical methods
  to avoid STDs. This can include avoiding risk

factors and using reliable preventive products/ services.

- Prevention of most prevalent STDs begins with changing risky sexual behaviors.
- Currently only Hep A & B and HPV can be prevented by vaccination.
- Post-exposure prophylaxis is yet another option available for several dreadful STDs such as HIV, Hep B, and gonorrhea.
- Suppressive therapy has promise and hope for people infected by HIV and HSV.
- People unwilling or unaware of condom use must be informed of the advantages and benefits.
- Limiting number of sex partners, safe sex practices, and partner selection options need to be stressed.
- Avoid sex with alcoholics and needle sharing drug addicts.
- Avoid sex with persons of unknown health/ STD status and commercial sex workers.

Primary care physicians and professionals in charge of STD clinics in the U.S. are well aware of most current practices and products available for control and prevention of STDs. When confronted with sexual health issues/ concerns visit the nearest clinic, talk to the doctor and have all your questions answered. Follow doctor's helpful suggestions as best as you can. Essential services and practices listed below come with instructions and follow up care.

- Accurate diagnosis followed by treatment. Symptoms for some STDs can be misleading therefore initial presumptive diagnosis must be routinely followed up by other definitive diagnostic procedures including reliable blood tests.
- Follow-up treatment and counseling services must be provided to all patients and their sex partners until everyone is cured and symptoms resolved.
- Patients must be warned of dangers and potential hazards of new infection and reinfection to self and sex partners. Abstinence until everyone is treated and cured is critical to all concerned.
- Identification of infected persons with no symptoms is a difficult task. Efforts must be made to reach out to people at risk. Current patient can be a useful resource to solicit such confidential information. Family and friends of patients can also greatly contribute to identify asymptomatic persons.

Pre-exposure immunization protects people for life. Viral STDs such as HPV and hepatitis (A&B) are preventable. Antiretroviral therapy (ART) has the potential to prevent HIV transmission and infection. Studies suggest that ART can significantly reduce risk for HIV. Risk for HSV transmission and acquisition can also be significantly reduced by antiviral suppressive therapy. Ask your doctor if it can work for you.

Post exposure prophylaxis (PEP) can substantially reduce risk for HIV and hepatitis B to victims of sexual assault. PEP is also available to victims of accidental and incidental exposure to several STDs.

Professional counseling, education, and accurate information are vital to prevent and control STDs. The method of choice should be convenient, safe, and above all practical to person's "life-style" needs. This guide has listed few methods for prevention and control of STDs. Your physician may offer choices and recommend method(s) that work best for you.

## 1. Abstinence:

- Most reliable method to remain free of STDs is abstinence from genital, oral, and anal sex. Person(s) committed to life - long monogamous relationship with uninfected partner can enjoy worry free, healthy sex life. Health conscious people can choose screening for common STDs prior courtship and anticipated long- term relationship.

- Abstinence is recommended for persons whose sex partner(s) are under treatment for any STD. Sex should be resumed only after every one infected is fully recovered.

- Abstinence from sexual activity is highly recommended for persons and their partners who have any signs of STIs. Sex should be resumed only upon professional advice.

## 2. Pre-exposure vaccination and prophylaxis:

- Currently two HPV vaccines (bivalent and quadrivalent) are available for males and females to prevent HPV infection. Genital warts and cervical cancer can be prevented for life: ask your doctor and protect yourself and your partner (s).
- Hepatitis A and B vaccines are recommended for all uninfected adults. Vaccines administered as recommended can protect recipients for life.
- For men with male sex partners (MSM) and injection drug- users (IDUs) hepatitis A and B vaccines are highly recommended.
- Hepatitis A and B vaccine has preventive benefits to HIV patients who have not yet been infected by hepatitis A and B.
- Research is underway to develop vaccines for other viral STDs such as HIV, HCV, and HSV.
- Persons suspecting acquiring STDs such as HIV, HSV, HAV, and HBV can opt for post-exposure prophylaxis. Vaccine, immunoglobulin or medications administered immediately after exposure can prevent viral transmission.

## 3. Male Condoms:

Three kinds of male condoms are available in the U.S. Condoms are used primarily to avoid pregnancy but used as directed can effectively prevent transmission of most common STDs including HIV. Condoms are classified as medical devices hence are subject to scrutiny by the U.S.

Food and Drug Administration (FDA). Currently available safe condoms are:

(a) Latex condoms manufactured in the U.S. are electronically tested for defects.
Condoms can occasionally break during sexual intercourse but condom failure rate is very low and rarely results in unintended pregnancy or STD transmission.

(b) Polyurethane or synthetic condom performs equal to latex device hence persons allergic to latex can substitute synthetic device for similar benefits.

(c) Natural or "lambskin" condom can prevent pregnancy but not viral STDs.

## 4. Female Condoms and Cervical Diaphragms:

(a) Female condom provides an effective barrier to common STDs including HIV. Female condom can be used if male condom is not available. Persons engaged in receptive anal intercourse should consider this device for protection against STDs and HIV.

(b) Diaphragm, yet another barrier device can protect against chlamydia, gonorrhea, and trichomoniasis. Protection against viral antigens cannot be totally relied upon diaphragm alone therefore consult your physician.

## 5. Condoms, Topical Microbicides, and N-9 Vaginal Spermicides:

Sexually active males and females resort to condoms and lubricating gels containing microbicides and spermicides to prevent common STDs and pregnancy. Some of these products have promise and potential in preventing HIV and other STDs but contain N-9, a spermicide. Frequent use of products containing N-9 is associated with increased risk for HIV transmission and urinary tract infection. N-9 can damage anogenital epithelium thus enabling transmission of bacteria and virus.

## 6. Contraception, Surgical Sterilization, and Hysterectomy:

Sexually active women who use oral contraception, have had hysterectomy, have intrauterine device (IUDs), or have been surgically sterilized may avoid pregnancy but not STDs. Healthcare providers should counsel women risk for common STDs and appropriate preventive procedures.

## 7. Male Circumcision:

Circumcised males are at much lower risk to acquire common STDs including HIV, HPV, and HSV. The world Health organization (WHO) and the Joint United Nations Programme on HIV/AIDS (UNAIDS) recommend male circumcision to prevent HIV and other STDs. In most developed countries circumcision is routinely performed upon birth of a male child. Poor and underdeveloped countries require resources in order to promote male circumcision and aggressively fight HIV/AIDS epidemic.

## 8. Teens and Adults in Prisons and Correctional Facilities:

Teens and adults entering correctional facilities and prisons in the U.S. have exceptionally high rate of STDs, especially hepatitis B, C, and HIV. Most criminals lodged in such facilities come from poor socio-economic status, live in cities, urban areas, and belong to ethnic or racial minorities. Risky sexual behaviors such as un-protected sex, multiple sex partners, commercial, and coerced sex are common among most people of such background. Most such men and women also known to abuse drugs and alcohol, self-treat, or get no treatment at all therefore fail to resolve STDs or other ailments promptly.

When infected incarcerated people leave detention facilities they too bring greater risk to the general population. The cycle continues unabated. In many states in the U.S. most correction facilities lack resources, skilled manpower, and above all programs to prevent transmission and spread of STDs. The program must involve initial testing, screening for common STDs/HIV, treatment, counseling, partner management, and follow-up.

Prisons and correctional facilities in most countries of the world fare no better than their U.S. counterparts. In most countries prisoners receive substandard healthcare (if any) and rarely quality treatment. Freed infected inmates therefore present a grave health risk to family, friends, and general public.

## STD Surveillance

Medical care and delivery system(s) in the U.S. is the envy of the world. Almost all communities in every state have offices managed by professional healthcare personnel. Well established procedures and guidelines to screen, test, and diagnose patient's concerns are in place. Critical information such as past history of STDs, sexual practices, sex partners, and treatment history is obtained from each patient in order to provide quality care, counseling, and partner management.

In the U.S., STD prevention and control procedures are designed to help individual needs: patients and victims of sexual assault and child abuse included. Victims are treated with dignity, compassion, counseled, and provided appropriate professional care. The customized special care and treatment consists of methods listed below.

- Women and young girls, victims of sexual assault or abuse have to cope with risk for STDs and pregnancy. Post exposure prophylaxis (PEP) for HIV and other common STDs are available in all such situations. Professional counseling and emergency contraception is provided upon request.
- Victims of sexual assault and abuse are provided specialized follow-up care and retesting for common STDs and HIV. Retesting can detect repeat infections even among asymptomatic people. This method has the potential to enhance prevention among victims' friends and family.
- Partner notification and management is a critical service to all patients. In the U.S., most communities offer such service. Partner management offers unique and important avenue to reach people who may be infected or about to be infected. The concept is designed to identify and reach infected persons promptly, and prevent/control spread of STDs and HIV. In many instances sex partners may be predators, MSM, and needle sharing drug addicts.

STDs such as HIV, chancroid, chlamydia, gonorrhea, and syphilis are reportable in every state in the U.S.
Reporting can be laboratory or provider based that may
vary from state to state. In most communities these reports
are protected by strict confidentiality guidelines. Most clinics and healthcare providers seek  information such as
medical history, symptoms, and identity of sex partner (s)
to comply with the law – it's in patient's best interest (and
obligation) to provide  list of  sex partners truthfully - all
such information will have tremendous impact in the control and prevention of all dreadful, even fatal diseases.

Most community health centers and hospitals treat,
manage, and counsel patients for sexually transmitted
diseases. Education, guidance, and support are also available along with treatment. You may be advised to change/
modify sexual behavior, drinking, drug, and other habits
to protect yourself and control the spread of STDs. Many
schools and public health centers with the help of local
health department offer educational programs for interested people - your local public library, hospital, Red Cross,
newspaper, and radio may have such information available
to you - just inquire.

Prevention of transmission and strategy to control the
spread of viral STDs such as HIV, herpes, hepatitis (B &
C), HPV, and others require much more effort. Many who
acquire viral STDs may look and feel healthy but asymptomatic. Unaware of their active infectious status, they may
transmit infection to susceptible people. Then it may be
too late. Viral STDs therefore is a true challenge for the
medical community. Education, counseling, more education, more counseling, and more of both to all sexually

active persons is the best and probably the only tool available to control the spread of viral STDs at this time. If you ever suspect contacting any STD see your physician immediately - any delay may cause great discomfort, inconvenience, financial drain and worse YOUR OWN LIFE! Few tips listed below may help.

- See your doctor if you or your partner (s) see/ feel any symptoms for STDs.
- Inform your sex partner (s) if you have any symptoms for STDs.
- Keep in mind that if you have any STD, your partner is also infected by it.
- Abstain until sex partner (s) and you are tested, completed treatment (if indicated) for STDs of concern, and free of infection therefore risk free.
- Risk to sex partner(s) can be minimized by safe sex practices as already described.

In the U.S., most communities offer compassionate care, counseling, and support for all who seek help. No matter where you reside look for the following in your local telephone directory, newspapers, public library, or media news bulletins.

- Health Department and Clinic
- Community services.
- Church and religious groups.
- Local Red Cross.
- Charitable organizations.

- Public and private libraries.
- Support groups with programs specially targeted to HIV/AIDS patients.
- Support/education programs for sexually active adults for all STDs.
- Alcoholics Anonymous.
- Drug Rehab centers.

For most current updates and health issues you may also contact:

1. Centers for Disease Control and Prevention (CDC) at www.cdc.gov
2. National Institute of Health (NIH) at www.nih.gov

# Abbreviations and Select Glossary

Abstinence: Self – restraint, usually refers to sex.

AIDS: acquired immune deficiency syndrome, condition caused by HIV.

Anoscopy: A procedure performed to examine inside wall of the anus.

Antibody: Protein produced by the immune system in response to foreign substances and pathogens such as bacteria, fungus, parasites, and virus.

Antigen: Surface (cell-wall) protein of pathogens that stimulates host's immune system into producing antibodies.

ART: Anti-retroviral therapy. Therapy refers to HIV.

Bacterium: A single celled organism (microbe) associated with infection. Many harmless and beneficial bacteria also exist.

Bisexual: A person who has sex with persons of same and opposite sex.

BV: Bacterial vaginosis.

Carrier: An infected person with or without symptoms who can transmit infection to others by association, sexual intimacy, and sharing needles.

CBC: Complete blood count.

CIN: Cervical intraepithelial neoplasia.

CLD: Chronic liver disease.

CSW: Commercial sex worker

Culture: A laboratory procedure used to grow and identify microbes such as bacteria, fungus, parasite, and virus.

DNA: Deoxyribonucleic acid.

Dysuria: Burning/pain associated with urination.

Ectopic Pregnancy: Implantation of fertilized egg outside the uterus usually in the fallopian tube.

EIA: Enzyme immunoassay.

ELISA: Enzyme linked immune-absorbent assay.

FDA: U.S. Food and Drug Administration.

FTA-ABS: Fluorescent treponemal antibody absorption test.

gG: Glycoprotein G.

HAART: Highly active antiretroviral therapy.

HAV: Hepatitis A virus.

HBsAg: Hepatitis B surface antigen.

HBV: Hepatitis B virus.

HCV: Hepatitis C virus.

HIV: Human immunodeficiency virus.

HPV: Human papillomavirus.

HR –HPV: High risk HPV.

HSV: Herpes simplex virus.

IDU: Injection drug use/user.

Ig: Immune globulin.

IgG: Immune globulin G.

IgM: Immune globulin M.

IM: Intramuscular

Immune System: A very complex body's defense mechanism that fights infection(s) and malignancies.

IUD: Intrauterine device – a medical device inserted into the uterus to prevent unwanted pregnancy.

KOH: Potassium hydroxide.

LGV: Lymphogranuloma venereum.

Lymph Node: Part of the immune system that consists of cell-clusters located around the body such as arm pits, groin, neck etc. Lymph nodes swell in response to infection, malignancy, and pain.

MAC Disease: Mycobacterium avium complex disease.

MRI: Magnetic Resonance Imaging.

MSM: Men who have sex with men.

Mucopurulent: Discharge produced in response to infection - mucous and pus.

N-9: Nonoxynol.

NAAT: Nucleic acid amplification test.

NGU: Non-gonococcal urethritis.

NNRTI: Non-Nucleoside Reverse Transcriptase Inhibitors.

NRTI: Nucleoside Reverse Transcriptase Inhibitors.

NtRTI: Nucleotide Reverse Transcriptase Inhibitors.

NSU: Nonspecific urethritis.

OSHA: Occupational Safety & Health Administration, U.S. Department of Labor.

OTC: Over- the - counter medications.

Pap smear test: A procedure to examine cervical cells for abnormalities, cell composition and cellular changes in order to detect or rule out cervical cancer.

PCR: Polymerase chain reaction.

PEP: Post-exposure prophylaxis.

PI: Protease Inhibitors.

PID: Pelvic Inflammatory Disease.

Prodrome: Symptoms indicating onset of an infection such as herpes outbreak.

Prophylactic: Medication(s) or devices prescribed to prevent infection.

RPR: Rapid plasma reagin test.

STD: Sexually Transmitted Disease.

STI: Sexually transmitted infection.

TCA: Trichloroacetic acid.

UTI: Urinary tract infection.

**VDRL:** Venereal Disease Research Laboratory test.
**VVC:** Vulvovaginal Candidiasis.
**WBC:** White blood count.
**WHO:** World Health Organization.
**WSW:** Women who have sex with women.

# Select References and Suggested Reading

1. Brooks, J.T., Kaplan, J.E., Holmes, K. K., et al: HIV-associated opportunistic infections – going, going, but not gone: the continued need for prevention and treatment guidelines; Clin. infect Dis: 48:609-611, 2009
2. Centers for Disease Control (CDC). Sexually transmitted diseases treatment guidelines, 2010. MMWR 59 (RR-12): 1-110.
3. CDC. Quadrivalent Human Papillomavirus Vaccine: Recommendations of the Advisory Committee on Immunization Practices (ACIP). MMWR 2007; 56 (No. RR- 2) 1-24.
4. CDC. FDA licensure of quadrivalent human papillomavirus vaccine (HPV4, Gardasil) for use in males and guidance from the Advisory Committee on Immunization Practices (ACIP). MMWR 2010; 59: 630 -2
5. CDC. FDA licensure of bivalent human papillomavirus vaccine (HPV-2, Cervarix) for use in females and updated HPV vaccination recommendations from the Advisory Committee on Immunization Practices (ACIP). MMWR 2010; 59: 626 – 9.
6. CDC. HIV/AIDS surveillance report, 2008, vol. 20, Atlanta, GA: US Department of Health and Human Services, Centers for Disease Control and Prevention; 2010.
7. CDC. Sexually Transmitted Disease Surveillance 2009. Atlanta, GA: US Department of Health and Human Services; November 2010.

8. CDC. Guidelines for prevention and treatment of opportunistic infections in HIV-infected adults and adolescents. MMWR 2009; 58(No.RR-4).

9. CDC. Recommendations for partner services programs for HIV Infection, syphilis, gonorrhea, and chlamydial infection. MMWR 2008; 57(No. RR-9): 1- 83.

10. CDC. Expedited Partner Therapy in the Management of Sexually Transmitted Disease. Atlanta, GA: US Department of Health and Human Services; 2006.

11. Eng, T. R., Butler, and W. T., eds: Committee on prevention and control of Sexually Transmitted Diseases, Institute of Medicine: The hidden epidemic: Confronting sexually transmitted diseases, Washington DC., 1997. National Academies Press. Washington, D.C.

12. Gilbert L, Alexander L, Grosshans JF, Jolley L. Answering frequently asked questions about HPV. Sex Transm Dis. 2003; 30 (3):193-194.

13. Goldsmith MR, Bankhead CR, Kehoe ST, Marsh G, Austoker J. Information and cervical screening: a qualitative study of women's awareness, understanding and information needs about HPV. J Med Screen. 2007; 14(1) 29-33.

14. Gupta R, Warren T, Wald A. Genital herpes. Lancet. 2007; 370: 2127-2137.

15. Handsfield, H. Hunter. Color atlas and synopsis of sexually transmitted diseases, 3rd ed. 2011. The McGraw-Hill Companies, Inc. New York, USA.

16. Mandell, Douglas, and Bennett's Principles and Practice of Infectious Diseases: eds: Mandell GL, Bennett JE, and Dolin r, 6th ed. 2005. Churchill Livingstone Philadelphia, PA.

17. Marr, Lisa. Sexually Transmitted Diseases, 2nd. ed. 2007. The Johns Hopkins University Press, Baltimore, MD. 21218 - 4363.

18. Minkin, Mary Jane, M. D. and Wright, Carol V., Ph.D. A Women's Guide to Sexual Health. Yale University Press Health and Wellness, 2003, 2005.

19. Moore, Elaine A. and Lisa M. Encyclopedia of Sexually Transmitted Diseases. McFarland, 2005.

20. Netter's Infectious Diseases eds: Elaine C. Jong, Dennis L. Stevens; Elsevier Saunders, 1600 John F. Kennedy Blvd. Ste 1800, Philadelphia, PA. 19103-2899.

21. Stanberry LR, and Bernstein DI, eds: Sexually Transmitted Diseases. Vaccines, Prevention and Control. Division of Infectious Diseases, Children's Hospital Medical Center, Cincinnati, Ohio, USA. Academic Press 2000.

22. U.S. Preventive Services Task Force. Screening for chlamydial infection: recommendation statement. Ann Intern Med 2007; 147: 128-34.

23. U.S. Preventive Task Force. Behavioral counseling to prevent sexually transmitted infections: recommendation statement. Ann Intern Med 2008; 149: 491-6.

24. Zenilman, J. M., and Moshen, S., eds: Sexually Transmitted Infections: Diagnosis, Management, and Treatment, 2012: Jones & Bartlet Learning, 40 Tall Pine Drive, Sudbury, MA 101776

# Author

Arthur D'Souza (Ph.D. 1973) owned and operated a successful clinical diagnostic laboratory (1977- 2000) in Cincinnati, Ohio. Prior to setting up Cincinnati Med-Lab, Dr. D'Souza served as a Laboratory Director providing technical consulting, quality control guidelines, routine operational, and logistic support to a large Independent Laboratory in upstate New York.

In 1973, soon after graduation Dr. D'Souza accepted Postdoctoral Research Associate position at Gamble Research Institute, Cincinnati, Ohio. He was part of Dr. Gilbert Schiff's research team that conducted public health projects in Infectious and Communicable Diseases of viral origin. During graduate and postgraduate studies Dr. D'Souza was employed as a Laboratory Technologist in several greater Cincinnati area hospital laboratories.

Dr. D'Souza is currently retired and resides in Cincinnati Suburb with wife Margaret. He enjoys outdoors and gardening.

Please share your comments and suggestions with Dr. D'Souza:

arthurdsouza43@gmail.com

arthurdsouza43@hotmail.com

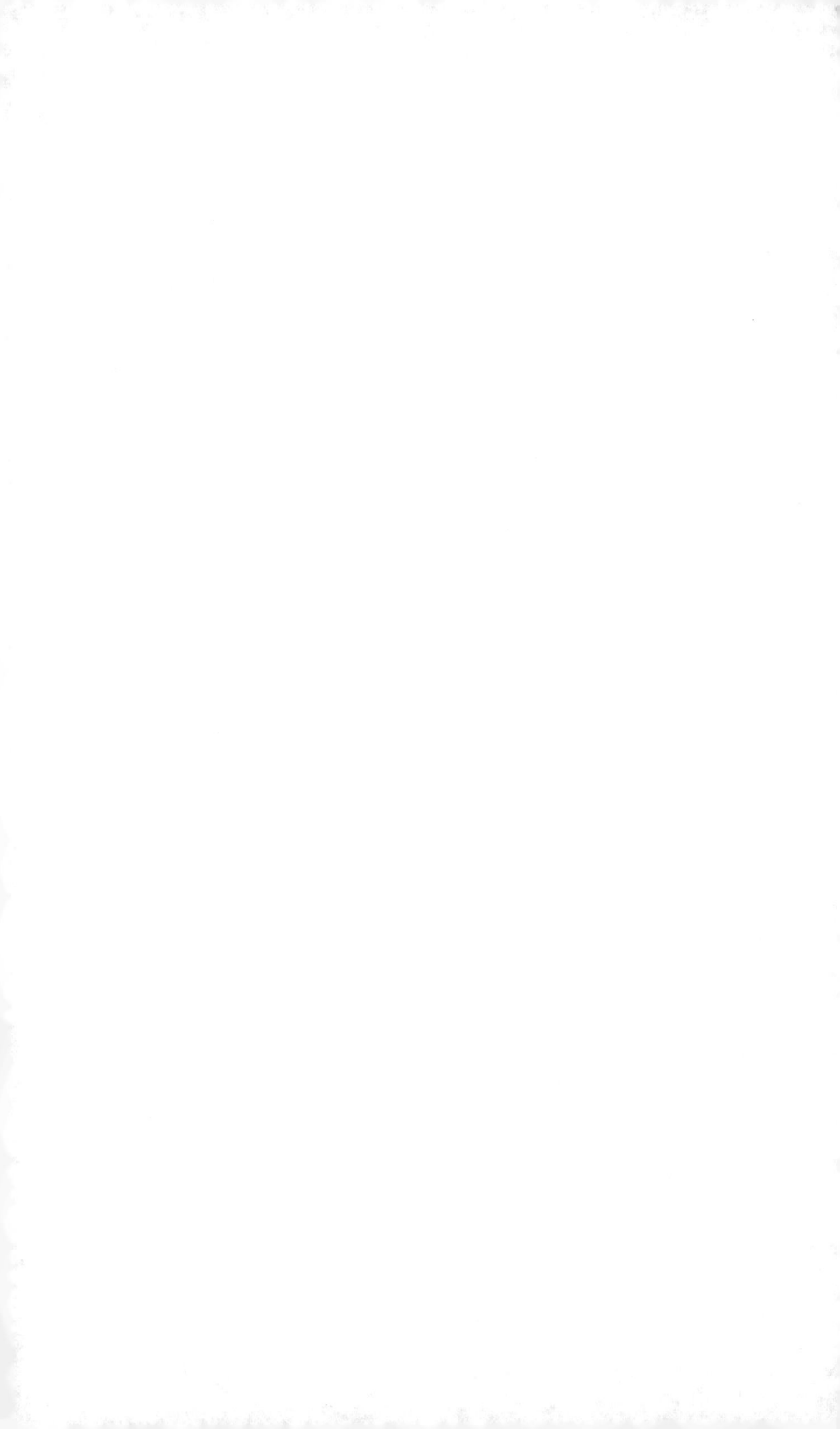

www.ingramcontent.com/pod-product-compliance
Lightning Source LLC
Chambersburg PA
CBHW070628290526
45790CB00001B/38